A Primer of Drug Action

A Series of Books in Psychology

Editors:
Richard C. Atkinson
Jonathan Freedman
Gardner Lindzey
Richard F. Thompson

Robert M. Julien

GOOD SAMARITAN HOSPITAL AND MEDICAL CENTER
Portland, Oregon

A Primer of Drug Action

Second Edition

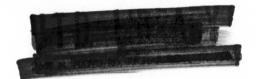

 W. H. FREEMAN AND COMPANY
San Fra

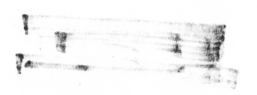

Library of Congress Cataloging in Publication Data

Julien, Robert M
  A primer of drug action.

  (A series of books in psychology)
  Bibliography: p.
  Includes index.
  1. Psychopharmacology. I. Title.
RM315.J75 1978   615'.78   77-13824
ISBN 0-7167-0053-0
ISBN 0-7167-0052-2 pbk.

Printed in the United States of America

10 9 8 7 6 5 4 3 2 1

Contents

Preface

Many books have been written about drugs. On the one hand there are the multitudes of popular books dealing with various aspects of drug abuse, books used in drug-education programs to try to discourage young people from experimenting with drugs. Many of these books have emphasized the moral, social, and physical degradation thought to result from drugs and they have often been laced with misinformation.

On the other hand there are the standard textbooks of pharmacology, that branch of science dealing with the study of drugs and their actions, which are intended for students of medicine, pharmacy, and other paramedical fields. These texts include the reference books written for professionals and graduate students in pharmacology. Such books assume an understanding of anatomy, physiology, biochemistry, and organic chemistry.

What was needed, I felt—and the response to the first edition of this book seems to have borne it out—was a drug-education book that was accurate, factual, and completely consistent. It had to be a book that was patterned after the classical pharmacology textbooks but written for people with little or no scientific background in biology, physiology, biochemistry, and related subjects. And it had to be free of professional jargon, so as not to confuse the general reader, yet not so lacking in content as to deter the student of science from reading it. Finally, I felt, it had to be written on the presumption that in many situations where the material might be presented the instructor might have only a limited knowledge of drugs and might lack the personal experiences of drugs shared by many of the students. In short, the information had to be scientifically correct yet comprehensible and relevant to the reader's life.

A drug may be broadly defined as any chemical substance that affects living processes. Obviously, this makes pharmacology quite an extensive subject. However, this book is restricted to those drugs commonly considered to be psychoactive and therefore subject to recreational use and abuse.

Both as a research neuropharmacologist working in the laboratory and as a physician working in clinics and hospitals, I find the study of drugs and their effects on the body, brain, and behavior fascinating. I hope that in this book I have made the subject also absorbing to readers.

ORGANIZATION OF THE BOOK

How has this book been organized so that it may be useful to audiences of such widely varying backgrounds as I outlined above? It seemed best to start with some of the principles of how drugs are handled by the body. Chapter 1, therefore, consists of a brief discussion of some of the general properties of drugs and the general principles by which drugs act in the body.

After this introductory chapter, I present material on psychoactive drugs, with extended discussion of the barbiturates, sedatives, alcohol, amphetamine and other stimulants, opiates, antipsychotics, psychedelics, and marijuana.

After the several chapters on psychoactive drugs, I have included a thought-provoking yet practical chapter on the processes of sexual reproduction, both male and female, and how they may be influenced by certain drugs such as the oral contraceptives. The pharmacology of antifertility drugs is also discussed and various alternatives to the use of drugs for the control of fertility and prevention of pregnancy are presented. I have found in my own courses on drugs that students are greatly interested in this topic.

The final chapter of the book presents a brief discussion of what has been called "drug abuse." Although this is a book about psychoactive drugs, it is not primarily a book on drug abuse. A colleague reviewing the chapter remarked that it was "somewhat embryonic" and could be easily expanded or padded. I have chosen not to do so, however, because I feel that once people have studied the pharmacology of these drugs, they can reach their own conclusions about the role of drugs in our society and I as an educator need not arrive at conclusions for them. The problem of drug misuse, as is pointed out, is not a problem of drugs but a problem of life and of people.

A word about the appendixes. They are designed to be useful. This book was not written to overwhelm the reader with biology, and so therefore a great deal of background material was placed in appendixes. It is there to be used by readers not familiar with neurophysiology and may be read at any appropriate time during treatment of the drug material. Indeed, for thorough and complete understanding of the chapters on specific drugs, the reader may want to cover the material on neurophysiology first. The book is written in such a manner, however, that this material is optional and not absolutely necessary. Chapter 1, for instance, may be augmented by the discussions in the appendixes of drug absorption and transport and the concept of a dose-response relationship. Appendixes I through III contain elementary yet comprehensive chapters on physiological psychology, the chemistry of synaptic transmission, elementary neurophysiology, and introductory neuroanatomy.

FEATURES OF THE NEW EDITION

There have been rapid developments in the area of psychoactive drugs, and they have necessitated this updated version from the original edition published in 1975. There is new material on the pharmacology of the benzodiazepines, the phenothiazines, marijuana, and the oral contraceptives. New sections have been added dealing with the pharmacology of the synthetic opiate narcotics, the narcotic antagonists, lithium, and phencyclidine. New sections have also been added on alcoholism, treatment and rehabilitation of the opiate user, and biological theories of psychosis. Finally, the bibliography has been updated and expanded.

ACKNOWLEDGMENTS

Since I feel that this book is somewhat unique in the pharmacological literature, I have been obliged to draw upon the expertise of many of my colleagues, and I would like to thank each of them for invaluable help. Certainly if this book is useful it would not have been so without the assistance of my colleagues, particularly Jack Elder, who reviewed the manuscripts for both editions. I would also like to thank Mrs. Beth Knudsen for her patience and assistance with the manuscript. Most importantly, I am most thankful to my wife, Judi, and my two sons, Robert and Scott, to whom I dedicated the first edition and who gave so generously that this could be written. Finally, I would like to dedicate this second edition to my former chairman and colleague, Henry W. Elliott, one of my strongest supporters and a leader in the science of pharmacology.

October 1977   Robert M. Julien, *M.D., Ph.D.*

A Primer of Drug Action

Chapter 1

Principles of Drug Action: How Drugs Affect the Body

When you seek relief from headache with an aspirin, social relaxation with alcohol, or any other drug-induced alteration of your physical or psychological state, the drug you use must somehow get from the external world into your body and ultimately to the specific site within the body or brain where it can exert its effect.

Simple though this may sound, transporting a drug from outside the body to its ultimate site of action is a complex process. The taking of a drug involves the absorption of that drug into the bloodstream, the distribution of the drug by the circulating blood to all regions of the body, the action of the drug itself, the eventual breakdown of the drug into an inactive compound, and finally the excretion of the drug. These processes are involved when *any* drug is taken, whether for medical or recreational purposes. Thus, let us briefly consider the physiological and biochemical processes involved.

DRUG ADMINISTRATION AND ABSORPTION

The terms *drug administration* and *drug absorption* refer to those mechanisms by which drugs are transported from the point of entry—stomach, intestine, or lungs—into the bloodstream. When administering any drug, one must be able to select a *route* of administration, a *dose* of the drug, and a *dosage form* (liquid, tablet, capsule, injection) that will place the drug at its site of action in a pharmacologically effective concentration and maintain this concentration for an adequate period of time.

Drugs are most commonly administered in four ways: *orally* (through the mouth), *rectally* (into the rectum), *parenterally* (by injection), and by *inhalation* through the lungs. Occasionally, drugs such as nasal decongestants and antiasthma drugs are administered through the *membranes of the mouth or nose.* A heart patient taking nitroglycerine, for instance, places the tablet under the tongue and the drug is absorbed into the bloodstream directly from the mouth. Cocaine, when sniffed, will be absorbed through the nose, because the powdered drug adheres to the membranes on the inside of the nose and is absorbed directly into the bloodstream. Let us consider these methods of administration and absorption in more detail.

Absorption by Mouth

Drugs are most commonly taken by mouth. To be administered orally, the drug must be soluble in stomach fluid, be carried to the intestine, penetrate the lining of the intestine, and pass into the bloodstream. Indeed, the degree to which a drug can be absorbed depends on its solubility (in stomach fluid) and permeability (through the lining of the intestine).

Alcohol, although taken by mouth, is absorbed slightly differently. Some is absorbed directly through the stomach into the bloodstream (a faster route of absorption, because the stomach contents need not first be emptied into the intestine). Indeed, if one drinks on an empty stomach, he may feel the effects of the alcohol very rapidly. If he drinks on a full stomach, the drug may pass into the intestine with the ingested food (into which it can dissolve), absorption is delayed, and its effects are slower to appear.

Drugs administered in liquid form, being already in solution, tend to be more rapidly absorbed than those given in tablet or capsule form. In solid form, the rate at which the drug dissolves becomes a limiting factor in its absorption. Occasionally, drugs are poorly manufactured and may fail to dissolve in the stomach. They may then pass through the intestine and be excreted in the feces without being absorbed into the body.

The dissolving and subsequent absorption of drugs into the bloodstream are fairly simple processes. The passage of a drug across the stomach lining, however, is more complicated (the process is explained in Appendix IV).

Although oral administration of drugs is widely used, it does have disadvantages. First, it may lead to occasional vomiting and stomach distress. Second, although it can be calculated how much drug is put into a tablet or capsule, it cannot always be accurately predicted how much of the drug will be absorbed into blood, owing to unexplained differences between individuals or differences in the manufacture of the drug. (Indeed, different brands of the same drug may be absorbed at widely differing rates.) Third, some drugs, such as procaine and insulin, when administered orally, are destroyed by the acid of the stomach or by the enzymes of the stomach and intestine before they can be absorbed. To be effective, such drugs must be administered by injection.

Absorption Through the Rectum

Although the primary route of drug administration is oral, some drugs are administered rectally (usually in a suppository) if the patient is vomiting, unconscious, or cannot swallow. However, absorption is often irregular, unpredictable, and incomplete, and many drugs irritate the membranes that line the rectum.

Absorption Through the Lungs

Administration by inhalation or injection are the more frequently used alternatives to administration by mouth and both methods bypass the gastrointestinal tract.

Drugs administered as gases penetrate the cell linings of the respiratory tract easily and rapidly. Anesthetic gases (such as nitrous oxide or ether) have small molecular sizes and high fat solubility. Therefore, these gases pass through the membranes of the lungs virtually as fast as they are inhaled and are absorbed promptly because of the close contact between the blood and the membranes of the lung. With very volatile substances (such as anesthetic gases), inhalation acts almost as fast as intravenous administration.

Despite our knowledge about the rapid absorption of gases through the lungs, very little is known about the pulmonary absorption of drugs other than those administered as gases. Cigarettes and marijuana are examples, since their active ingredients are not gases but particles carried in the smoke. Although many drugs *appear* to be absorbed readily when inhaled as sprays, aerosols, smoke, or dust, knowledge of the extent and rate of absorption is incomplete. However, from hundreds of years of experience with nicotine, opium, and marijuana, it is clear that inhalation is an effective mode of administration.

It is also becoming quite well known that inhalation of substances that are not volatile, such as tars, which are abundant in inhaled cigarette smoke, can injure the sensitive tissues of the lung. Lung cancer, which can be induced by long-term inhalation of cigarette smoke, is thought to be fatal in approximately 91 percent of cases and is estimated to result in 72,000 deaths a year in the United States. It is not yet known whether untoward effects will be produced by long-term inhalation of smoke obtained from marijuana or opium, even though current evidence indicates that bronchitis can be induced. Few Americans smoke either marijuana or opium anywhere nearly as heavily as do thousands who smoke cigarettes, and so lung tissue is less exposed.

Even if the frequency of marijuana smoking increases, lung damage is considered less likely. Several studies conducted in both Western and Eastern cultures indicate that even long-term, frequent smoking of marijuana and opium produces only minor pathological alterations in lung structure or function. This topic is discussed at length in Chapter 9. As a general rule, however, because of the ultrasensitivity of the lung tissue to foreign substances, administration of drugs by inhalation probably should not be exploited.

Absorption by Injection

Administration of drugs by injection can be *intravenous* (directly into a vein), *intramuscular* (directly into a muscle), or *subcutaneous* (just under the skin). Each of these avenues has its advantages and disadvantages, but some features are shared by all. In general, administration by injection produces a more prompt response than is obtainable by oral administration because absorption is more rapid after injection. More accurate dosage is attained with injections since the destruction of drugs in the gastrointestinal tract is avoided and the unpredictable processes of absorption through the stomach lining are bypassed.

Administration by injection, however, has several drawbacks. First, because of the rapid rate of absorption (since the absorption processes through the stomach and intestine are bypassed), there is often little time to respond to an unexpected drug reaction or accidental overdose. Second, administration by injection requires sterile conditions. The result of unsterile techniques may be so drastic as to lead to infectious disease or abscesses. Third, the injection itself may be painful, and once a drug is administered it cannot be recalled.

An overdose of an orally administered drug may be counteracted by the induction of vomiting if the drug has not yet been completely absorbed into the bloodstream. In a hospital emergency room, a conscious patient who has orally ingested a large dose of barbiturates in a suicide attempt may be induced to vomit any undissolved tablets or capsules or any unabsorbed (although dissolved) drug. If the patient is *unconscious,* however, vomiting is usually *not* induced, as the vomitus may be inhaled into the lungs, so a tube is passed into the stomach and the drug is washed out.

INTRAVENOUS ADMINISTRATION

In intravenous (abbreviated i.v.) injection, a drug is introduced directly into the bloodstream. This technique avoids all the variabilities of oral absorption, and the drug is placed in the circulation with minimum delay. In addition, the dose of the drug may be controlled. The injection can be made slowly and it can be stopped instantaneously if untoward effects develop. Finally, the intravenous route permits the greatest accuracy in drug dosage, allows one to give large volumes of solution over a long period of time, and enables one to administer solutions that can irritate the veins, since, when given slowly, these become diluted in a large volume of fluid (the blood).

The intravenous route has several severe drawbacks, however. First, it is the most dangerous of all avenues of drug administration because of the speed of onset of pharmacological action, which is faster than that of intramuscular or subcutaneous injection. Second, if a normally safe dose is given too rapidly, catastrophic and life-threatening effects (such as collapse of respiration or of heart function) may result. Third, allergic reactions to the drug may be mild when the drug is administered orally but may be extremely severe when the same drug is administered intravenously. Fourth, drugs that are not soluble in the blood or drugs dissolved in oily liquids may not be given intravenously because of the danger of blood clots forming.

Finally, infection by bacterial contaminants is a continuous danger, and infectious diseases or abscesses may be induced unless sterile techniques are employed.

INTRAMUSCULAR ADMINISTRATION

Drugs injected into skeletal muscle (usually in the arm or the buttocks) are generally absorbed fairly rapidly. Absorption of a drug from muscle is more rapid than absorption of the same drug from the stomach but is slower than when the drug is administered intravenously. The absolute rate of absorption of a drug from muscle depends on the rate of the blood flow to that muscle, the solubility of the drug, and the volume of the injection.

In general, most of the precautions that apply to intravenous administration apply to intramuscular injection. However, drugs intended for intramuscular administration should not usually be given intravenously, and one must be careful to avoid hitting a blood vessel when inserting a needle into muscle. Such an accident would result in inadvertent i.v. injection.

SUBCUTANEOUS ADMINISTRATION

Absorption of drugs that have been injected under the skin (subcutaneously) is quite rapid. The exact rate depends mainly on the ease with which the drugs penetrate the walls of the blood vessels and the rate of the blood flow through the skin. Irritating drugs should not be injected subcutaneously since they may produce severe pain and local tissue damage. The usual precautions to maintain sterility apply.

Self-administration of any drug by injection is to be discouraged except in certain circumstances (such as the injection of insulin by a diabetic) where oral administration is ineffective or when the drug is being taken therapeutically under a physician's direction. The risks associated with injection of a drug (risks of infection, overdose, allergic responses, and so forth) are often far greater than those associated with the oral administration of the same drug.

DISTRIBUTION OF DRUGS THROUGHOUT THE BODY

Once it is absorbed into the bloodstream, a drug is distributed throughout the body by the circulation of the blood. However, even after the drug reaches the bloodstream, it must still pass across various barriers in order to reach its site of action. Only a very small portion of the total amount of a drug in the body at any one time is in direct contact with the specific cells that produce the pharmacological action of the drug. Most of the drug is to be found in areas of the body remote from the drug's site of action. In the case of psychoactive drugs (drugs that alter mood or behavior as a result of their effect on the central nervous system), most of the drug is to be found outside the brain and is therefore not directly contributing to the pharmacological effect.

In most discussions on psychoactive drugs, writers discuss only that amount of drug that is in the brain actively producing the pharmacological and psychological effects. Yet it is the total amount of drug in the body that governs the movements of the drug through the tissues of the body and its ultimate disappearance from the body, and thus determines both the length of time and the intensity of the drug's effect.

Distribution of Drugs by Blood

Each minute the heart pumps approximately 5 liters (1 liter = 2.1 pints) of blood. Since the total amount of blood in the circulatory system is only about 6 liters, the entire blood volume circulates in the body about once per minute. Once a drug is absorbed into the blood, it is quite rapidly (usually within this 1-minute circulation time) distributed throughout the circulatory system.

A schematic diagram of the circulatory system is presented in Figure 1.1. Blood returning to the heart from the veins is first pumped into the pulmonary (lung) circulation system where, in the lungs, carbon dioxide is removed from the blood and replaced by oxygen. The oxygenated blood then returns to the heart and is pumped into the great artery (the aorta). From here, blood flows into the smaller arteries and finally into the capillaries, where nutrients (and drugs) are exchanged between the blood and the cells of the body.

To perform this exchange, the body has an estimated 10 billion capillaries having a total surface area of more than 200 square meters. Probably no single functioning cell of the body is more than between 20 and 30 microns away from a capillary (1 micron = 0.0004 inch). A discussion of the structure and function of the capillary is presented below. After blood passes through the capillaries, it is collected by the veins, through which it returns to the heart to circulate again.

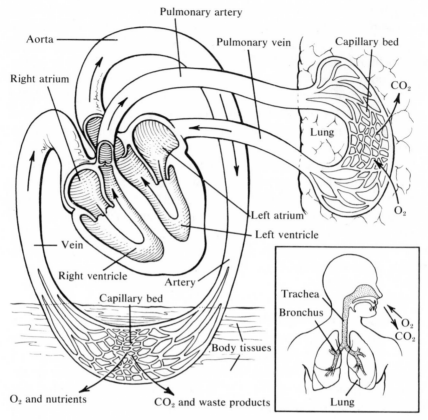

Figure 1.1. The heart and circulatory system. Blood returning from the body tissues to the heart via the veins passes through the right atrium into the right ventricle and, with the contraction of the heart, is pumped into the arteries leading to the lungs. In the lungs, carbon dioxide (CO_2) is lost and replaced by oxygen (O_2). This oxygenated blood returns to the heart through the left atrium, is pumped out of the left ventricle into the aorta, and is carried to the body tissues, where oxygen and nutrients are exchanged in the capillary beds. Oxygen and nutrients are supplied to the body tissues through the walls of the capillaries; CO_2 and other waste products are returned to the blood. The CO_2 is eliminated through the lungs, and the other waste products are excreted through the kidneys.

Thus, drugs are fairly evenly distributed throughout this 6 liters of blood. The normal, lean, 150-pound man, however, contains approximately 41 liters of water (58 percent of the total body weight is composed of water). Therefore, if 41 liters represents the total body water and 6 liters of this represents the volume of the circulating blood, the remaining 35 liters of water must be in the body tissues. However, this water is not isolated from the blood, for fluids (and drugs) are transferred between the blood and the body fluids in and around the cells of the body. Thus, drugs are diluted not only by the blood, but also by body water, since virtually all drugs can move out of the bloodstream and into the fluid that closely surrounds the cells of the body tissues. If the drug is capable of penetrating the cells, it will be further diluted by the intracellular fluids.

In addition to solubility, there is another factor that often limits the distribution of a drug in the body. Large amounts of many drugs may actually become bound firmly to proteins contained in the blood. Since blood proteins (albumin, for example) are quite large and thus are unable to leave the bloodstream, a drug that is bound to protein would be confined within the blood vessels. Unable to leave the bloodstream, such a drug is prevented from reaching the cells of the body tissues. The confinement of a drug within the blood vessels might appear to render it useless. Indeed, if the drug's site of action is outside the blood vessels (in the brain, for example), its binding to blood proteins would decrease its effectiveness. The more common situation, however, is that only small amounts of a drug are bound to blood proteins and the distribution of a drug may be more general, that is, throughout the body. In time, alcohol, for example, may be found in equal concentrations throughout all the body water.

Unequal distribution among body water compartments is illustrated for three drugs in Figure 1.2. After being absorbed from the stomach and into the bloodstream, drug 1 is bound almost completely to protein and is confined to the bloodstream. Drug 2 is not bound to blood proteins and easily passes out of the bloodstream into tissue fluid, but is unable to pass into cells and therefore does not have access to the fluid inside them. Drug 3 is a compound that easily passes out of the bloodstream and readily penetrates cell membranes into the fluid inside. An example of this last drug is thiopental (Pentothal), a commonly used anesthetic, which induces anesthesia within a matter of seconds when injected intravenously. Thiopental is extremely soluble in the fat of cell membranes, so it can rapidly leave the bloodstream and pass into cells in the brain, where it quickly depresses the brain and abolishes consciousness.

Body Membranes that Affect Drug Distribution

The absorption and distribution of drugs are affected by various types of membranes in the body. The four types of membranes that seem to be most important to the discussion are those of (1) the cell walls, (2) the walls of the capillary vessels of the circulatory

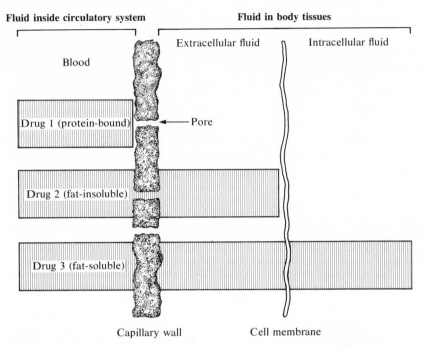

Figure 1.2. Distribution of three hypothetical drugs into different body compartments. *Drug 1* is bound to blood proteins; *drug 2* is unbound, soluble in water but insoluble in fat; *drug 3* is unbound and soluble in both water and fat. Note that *drug 1* is largely restricted to the bloodstream, *drug 2* is distributed in the blood and in the fluid outside the body cells, and *drug 3* is distributed through all the body compartments and readily passes into the brain, easily crossing the blood-brain barrier.

system, (3) the blood-brain barrier (a barrier that affects the passage of drugs into the brain), and (4) the placental barrier. Let us consider each of these.

CELL MEMBRANES

In order to be absorbed from the intestine or gain access to the interior of a cell, a drug has to penetrate the cell membranes. What, then, is known of the structure and properties of such membranes that determine their permeability to drugs? The generalized picture that has emerged from chemical, physiological, and electron micrograph studies is represented in Figure 1.3. The characteristic feature of the cell membrane appears to be a bimolecular sandwich of fat molecules coated by a protein layer on each surface, as two slices of bread (the protein) would enclose two slices of cheese (the fat layers). The total thickness of this membrane is about 80 angstroms. (The angstrom, which is abbreviated Å, is equal to 0.0001 micron or 0.00000004

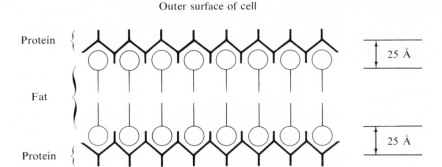

Figure 1.3. Structure of the cell membrane. The inner and outer layers of the cell membrane consist primarily of proteins with molecules of fat sandwiched between.

inch.) This protein and fat membrane provides a barrier that is permeable to some drug molecules and impermeable to others. Only drugs that are soluble in fat can pass through such a membrane.

In addition to this layered structure of protein and fat, the membrane appears to contain small holes or pores (about 8 Å in diameter) that permit the passage of small, water-soluble molecules, such as alcohol and water itself. These cellular barriers (as hindrances to the absorption and distribution of drugs) are important for the passage of drugs from the stomach and intestine into the bloodstream, from the fluid that closely surrounds tissue cells to the interior of cells, from interior of cells back into body water, and from the urinary system back into the bloodstream. Most drugs are too large to penetrate the small pores and, thus, most water-soluble, fat-insoluble drugs cannot pass through the cellular barriers. (Appendix IV offers an expanded discussion of the properties of drugs that determine their relative solubilities in cell membranes.)

BLOOD CAPILLARIES

As we have already discussed, drug molecules are distributed throughout the body by means of the circulation of blood. Within a minute or so after a drug enters the bloodstream, it is distributed fairly evenly through the bloodstream. However, most drugs are not confined to the bloodstream because they are exchanged back and forth across the blood capillaries.

Figure 1.4 is a cross-sectional diagram of a capillary. Capillaries are tiny cylindrical tubes with walls formed by a thin, unicellular layer of cells tightly packed together and surrounded (for structural rigidity) by a thin "basement" membrane. Between the cells are minute passageways (pores) connecting the interior of the tube (the capillary) with the exterior (the body tissues). These pores have a diameter of between 90 and 150 Å and are larger than most drug molecules. Since it is only in the capillaries that drugs are exchanged between blood and body cells, the capillaries must be small (to bring water and essential body nutrients into close contact with the surrounding cells) and numerous (10 billion, it has been estimated).

Because most drugs are smaller than the pores, drug molecules are able to pass out of the capillaries into surrounding tissue with only minimal difficulty. As a result, most drugs reach the cells of most body tissues within a fairly short time, limited primarily by the rate of blood flow to the tissue. Therefore, in the transport of drug molecules out of blood capillaries and into tissues (and conversely from tissues back into the blood through the capillaries), it does not matter whether a drug is soluble in fat since the membrane pores are large enough for even fat-insoluble drug molecules to penetrate. These drug molecules traverse the capillary membrane at a rate roughly proportional to the difference in concentration of the drug on either side of the capillary membrane; that is, the higher the concentration of the drug in the blood and the lower the concentration in the tissues, the faster the drug diffuses out of the capillary.

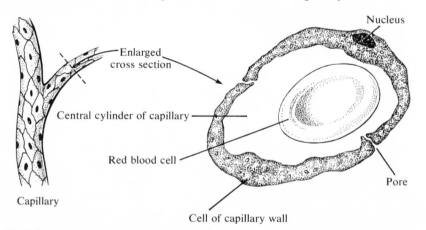

Figure 1.4. Cross section of a blood capillary. Within the capillary are the fluids, proteins, and cells of the blood, including the red blood cells. The capillary itself is made up of cells that completely surround and define the central cylinder (or lumen) of the capillary. Water-filled pores form channels allowing communication between the lumen and the fluid outside the capillaries.

These pores in the capillary membrane, however, are sufficiently small that the red blood cells and the blood proteins are largely confined to the bloodstream. Thus, the only drugs that do not readily penetrate capillary membranes are those rare drugs that are proteins and those that are bound to blood proteins. Since significant amounts of many drugs may be bound to blood protein and since these proteins do not readily diffuse across the capillary membrane, this bound fraction of drug is essentially trapped in the bloodstream and will not diffuse from the blood into the tissues. If a drug is capable of leaving the capillaries readily, its concentration in the blood will decline extremely rapidly and the drug might have both a rapid onset and a short duration of action.

The rate at which drug molecules enter specific tissues of the body depends upon two factors: the rate of blood flow through the tissue, and the ease with which drug molecules pass through the capillary membranes. Because blood flow is greatest to the brain and much poorer to the bones, joints, and fat deposits, drug distribution, everything else being equal, would follow a similar pattern. However, some capillaries (such as those in the brain) have special structural properties that may limit further the diffusion of a drug into the brain.

THE BLOOD-BRAIN BARRIER

The passage of drugs into the central nervous system is a special aspect of cellular penetration and is one example of the *unequal* distribution of drugs. The brain constitutes only 2 percent of the body weight and yet, under resting conditions, it receives 16 percent of the blood pumped by the heart. Thus, the brain is one of the body organs most richly supplied with blood. The average rate of blood flow to the brain is approximately 10 times that to resting muscles. Since the distribution of drugs to the various areas of the body is largely dependent upon the blood flow to the tissues, one might predict that drugs would pass very rapidly from blood to brain. Indeed, some compounds do reach the brain quickly (as in the thiopental example), but many drugs (penicillin, for example) enter brain tissue only slowly, if at all.

This decreased permeability of the capillaries of the brain has a structural basis (see Figure 1.5). Whereas, in most of the rest of the body, pores are present in the capillary membranes, the brain capillaries are tightly joined together and covered on the outside by a fatty, footlike sheath that arises from a nearby cell, an astrocyte. Thus, a drug leaving the capillaries in the brain has to traverse not only the

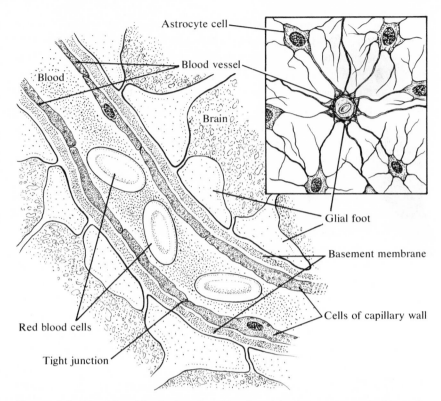

Figure 1.5. The blood-brain barrier. Blood and brain are separated both by capillary cells packed tightly together and by a fatty barrier called the glial sheath, which is made up of extensions (glial feet) from nearby astrocyte cells *(see inset)*. A drug diffusing from blood to brain must move through the cells of the capillary wall, because there are tight junctions rather than pores between the cells, and must then move through the fatty glial sheath.

capillary cell wall itself (since there are no pores to pass through) but also the membranes of the astrocyte cells in order to reach the cells in the brain. Such a structure tends, therefore, to limit the entry of many drugs into the brain. This decreased permeability of the capillaries in the brain to some substances is frequently described by the term *blood-brain barrier*. This term is widely used and is useful for distinguishing drugs that can penetrate the brain from those that cannot.

THE PLACENTAL BARRIER

Among all the membrane systems of the body, the placenta is unique. It separates two distinct human beings with differing genetic compositions, physiological responses, and sensitivities to drugs. The fetus obtains essential nutrients and eliminates metabolic waste products through the placenta without depending on its own organs, many of which are not yet functioning. This dependence of the fetus on the mother, however, places the fetus at the mercy of the placenta when foreign substances (such as drugs) appear in the mother's blood.

Pregnant women in the United States regularly take an average of four prescription drugs and many other drugs purchased without prescriptions, and they have an undetermined exposure to potentially toxic substances in food, cosmetics, household chemicals, and the general environment. The extent to which these latter substances affect the fetus is not yet known.

The effects of drugs on the fetus are of two major types. First, early in pregnancy, when the limbs and organ systems are being formed, drugs may induce structural abnormalities *(teratogenesis)*. The most dramatic example of a teratogenic compound was thalidomide, a tranquilizer marketed in several countries in the early 1960s, which, when given to women in the fifth through seventh weeks of pregnancy, produced a high incidence of abnormal growth of the limbs in the fetus. Second, later in pregnancy and during delivery, drugs may induce respiratory depression in the newborn baby because it is unable to metabolize or excrete them.

Schematic representations of the placental network, which transfers substances between mother and fetus, are shown in figures 1.6 and 1.7. In general, the mature placenta consists of a network of vessels and pools of maternal blood into which protrude treelike or fingerlike villi (projections) containing the blood capillaries of the fetus (Figure 1.7). Oxygen and nutrients move from the mother's blood to that of the fetus, while carbon dioxide and other waste products move from the fetal to the maternal blood.

The membranes separating fetal blood from maternal blood in the intervillous space resemble, in their general permeability, cell membranes found elsewhere in the body. Fat-soluble substances diffuse across readily, while fat-insoluble substances diffuse less well. This is of interest since late in pregnancy and at the time of delivery most anesthetic liquids and gases and most pain-relieving agents penetrate both the blood-brain barrier and placenta very readily.

Anesthetics and narcotic analgesics may be found in fairly high concentrations in the newborn infant. We are all aware of stories about the occurrence of withdrawal symptoms in infants born of addicted mothers, stories that make it clear that morphine and other narcotics have free access to, and an effect upon, the fetus during pregnancy. Tranquilizing and sedating drugs also cross the placenta

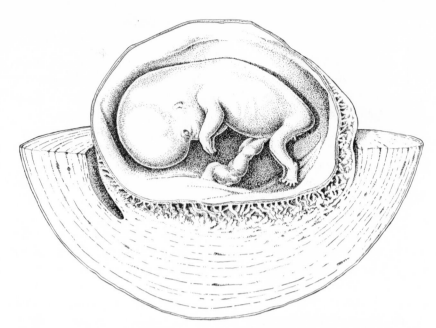

Figure 1.6. Placenta, embryo, and section through part of uterus. [Redrawn from W. J. Hamilton, J. D. Boyd, and H. W. Mossman, *Human Embryology: Prenatal Development of Form and Function* (Baltimore: Williams & Wilkins, 1962), fig. 86, p. 85. Courtesy of Professors Hamilton, Boyd, and Mossman and Mr. Heffer.]

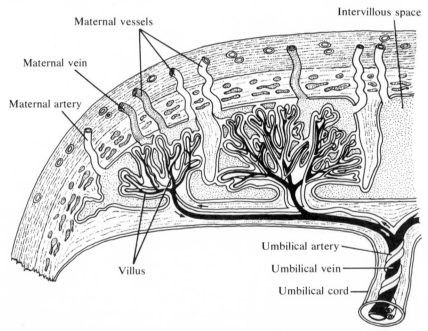

Figure 1.7. Placental network separating the blood of mother and fetus. [From C. M. Goss, ed., *Gray's Anatomy of the Human Body,* 29th ed. (Philadelphia: Lea and Febiger, 1973), fig. 2-51, p. 40.]

quite readily. The blood levels of a barbiturate administered intravenously to mothers in labor are plotted in Figure 1.8. The blood concentrations of the drug were determined in both maternal blood and fetal blood. You can see from this figure that significant amounts of the barbiturate are distributed to the infant and that, about 10 minutes after the injection, blood levels in the mother and in the newborn baby are almost identical.

To date, data are not available about a possible relation between the extent of drug use at delivery and the overall infant mortality. It is clear, however, that infants of mothers who are delivered under deep anesthesia are often less active than those delivered without benefit of drugs or with only small doses of depressants or narcotics and are physically and mentally depressed for the next 24 hours. The situation is further compounded by the fact that newborn babies, especially premature infants, have a very limited capacity to metabolize and excrete the drugs after delivery. To date, studies have not been conducted on the effects of either single doses or repeated doses of a drug on the fetus. Until details of these effects are known, the

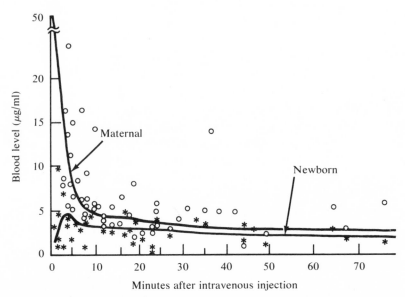

Figure 1.8. Effect of barbiturate on mothers in labor. Blood levels of secobarbital in mothers and their newborn infants after intravenous administration of the drug to the mothers. Each point represents one subject (*circles,* mothers; *asterisks,* infants). [From B. Roote, E. Eichner, and I. Sunshine, "Blood Secobarbital Levels and Their Clinical Correlation in Mothers and Newborn Infants," *American Journal of Obstetrics and Gynecology* 81 (1961): 948.]

fetus will continue to be treated with its mother in a rather haphazard manner, often inappropriately and sometimes with tragic results. The effects of drugs on the fetus is discussed further later in the chapter.

THE DRUG RECEPTOR AND THE MYTH OF THE "MAGIC BULLET"

Before producing a change in the functioning of a cell, which then leads to a change in body function or behavior, a drug must physically interact with one or more constituents of the cell. The cell component directly involved in this initial action of a drug is usually termed its *receptive substance* or, more simply, the drug *receptor*. It has been concluded from many years of pharmacological research that drugs must somehow interact with this receptor material in the cell before the drug can act and that certain small patches of the cell with special aptitudes or properties may give rise (when occupied by drug) to a chain of events that results in a detectable response. Thus, occupation of a receptor by a drug leads to a change of the functional properties of the cell.

A characteristic of the drug receptor is its high (but not absolute) degree of specificity for a drug molecule. What may appear to be a slight or insignificant variation in the chemical structure of a drug may greatly alter the intensity of the cell's response to the drug. For example, amphetamine and methamphetamine are both powerful stimulants of the central nervous system. They differ chemically only very slightly, but the change is such that methamphetamine is much more potent and, at equal doses of both drugs, produces much greater behavioral stimulation. Both drugs probably affect the same receptor in the brain, but for some reason, methamphetamine exerts a much more powerful action on that receptor.

It has been postulated that the drug molecule with the "best fit" to the receptor will elicit the most response from the cell. Thus, methamphetamine might "fit" the receptor better than amphetamine does. It is currently thought that the cellular response that follows the attachment of a drug to the receptor is followed by a change in the conformation of the cell membrane—a change that is thought to alter the cellular behavior and ultimately brain or body function.

In the television cartoon-advertisements for analgesic tablets, we see the compound being taken orally, dissolving in the stomach, being absorbed into the bloodstream, and then being rapidly (some more rapidly than others, according to the commercial message) distributed exclusively to the receptors (with hammers, pistons, lightning bolts, and so on) in the brain, which are immediately depressed so that the headache magically disappears. Thus, even in this day and age, a drug is often promoted as being some type of "magic bullet," which, upon being swallowed, immediately knows where its receptor is, streaks to that receptor, and in some mysterious way exerts its effect.

This idea of a drug's being selectively distributed to a very small area of the body is, of course, false. Subject to the physical and chemical factors discussed above, drugs are distributed through the body fairly evenly. There is no such thing as a magic bullet that somehow affects a specific target organ. Selectivity of drug action is more a function of the location of the drug receptors, the strength of the drug's attachment to the receptor, and the consequences of the interaction between drug and receptor than it is a property of selective distribution of the drug.

TERMINATION OF DRUG ACTION

Drug action may terminate even though the drug is still present in the body. For example, the anesthetic agent thiopental, because of its high fat solubility, penetrates the brain and produces unconsciousness within a few seconds. The duration of unconsciousness is quite short (the patient awakens within 5 or 10 minutes) because thiopental (being so soluble in fat) is rapidly removed from the brain and transported to fatty deposits in the body. Even though the patient is awake, he or she is not completely "normal," because small amounts of thiopental are still present in the blood and brain. Most of the drug is stored in muscle and fat awaiting metabolism and excretion.

Thiopental is somewhat an exception rather than the rule. Usually, in order to be removed from its site of action and from the bloodstream, a drug must be metabolized by the liver and excreted from the body by the kidneys. Thus, to complete our discussion of the body's response to drugs, we should describe those processes by which drugs are eliminated from the body.

Elimination of Drugs by the Kidneys

The kidneys are the main excretory organs of the body. There are three other channels for excreting waste substances and drugs— the lungs, the skin, and the intestine—but these are less important. (They are discussed briefly later in this chapter.)

Physiologically, the kidneys perform two major functions: first, they excrete most of the products of body metabolism (including drugs), and second, they closely regulate the levels of most of the substances found in body fluids. The kidneys are a pair of bean-shaped organs (see Figure 1.9), each a little smaller than a fist and weighing about a quarter of a pound. They lie at the rear of the abdominal cavity at the level of the lower ribs.

The outer portion of the kidney is made up of some two million functional units called nephrons (Figure 1.10). Each unit consists of a knot of capillaries (the glomerulus) through which blood flows from the renal artery to the renal vein. This glomerulus is surrounded by the opening of the nephron (Bowman's capsule) into which fluid flows as it filters out of the capillaries. Pressure of the blood in the glomerulus causes fluid to leave the capillaries and flow into Bowman's capsule, from which it flows through the tubules of the kidney and finally into a duct that collects fluid from several nephrons. This fluid from the collecting ducts is eventually passed through the ureters and into the urinary bladder, which is periodically emptied.

The basic function of the kidney is to maintain proper internal environment, and in doing so it rids the blood of unwanted substances as it passes through. Substances that must be excreted include the products of body metabolism and sodium, potassium, and chloride, which accumulate in the body in excess quantities. The kidney must also be capable of conserving water, sugar, and the necessary quantities of sodium, potassium, and chloride. The kidney rids the blood of unwanted substances and retains ingredients essential to the body,

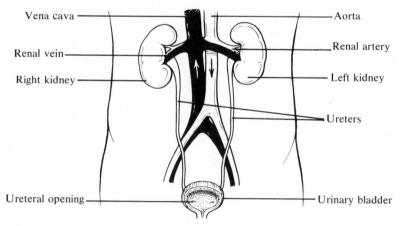

Figure 1.9. The architecture of the kidneys.

as follows: First, a large portion of the blood, usually about one-fifth of it, is filtered into the tubules of the kidney. Left behind in the bloodstream are blood cells, proteins, and a small amount of fluid. As the filtered fluid flows through the kidney tubules, the unwanted substances, failing to be reabsorbed into the bloodstream through the walls of the cells lining the tubules, pass into the urinary bladder for excretion later. Substances to be conserved are reabsorbed from the kidney into the bloodstream when they pass through the walls of the cells lining the tubules.

Since drugs are small particles dissolved in the blood, they, too, are usually filtered into the kidneys and then reabsorbed back into the bloodstream. Water is reabsorbed from the tubules into the bloodstream to a much greater extent than are most drugs, so the drugs become more concentrated inside the nephrons than they are in the blood. Since substances tend to move from areas of high concentration to areas of low concentration, drugs move out of the kidney

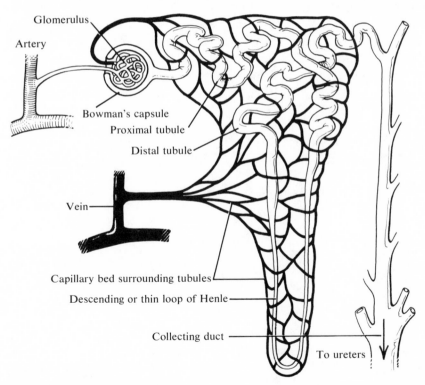

Figure 1.10. A nephron within a kidney. Note the complexity of the structure and the intimate relation between the blood supply and the nephron. Each kidney is composed of more than a million such nephrons.

back into the bloodstream. Thus, the kidney, working alone, is simply insufficient for the task of eliminating drugs from the body.

How, then, is the kidney able to function in the elimination of drugs from the body? In order for the body to hasten the urinary excretion of a drug, the drug must somehow be prevented from being reabsorbed from the urine into the bloodstream. The drug must be changed by metabolic processes in the body into a compound that is less fat soluble and therefore less capable of being reabsorbed. This process of converting fat-soluble drugs into water-soluble metabolites that can be excreted by the kidney is carried out by the liver (Figure 1.11). Usually (but not always) this process of metabolism also *decreases* the pharmacological activity of the drug. Thus, even though a metabolite might persist in the body (awaiting excretion), it would usually be pharmacologically inactive and would not produce the effects of the parent drug.

The exact mechanisms in the liver that result in chemical alterations in the structures of drugs is beyond the scope of our discussion, but suffice it to state that the reactions are carried out by a special system of enzymes in the liver cells. Many psychoactive drugs have the ability to *increase* the *rate* at which this enzyme system metabolizes a variety of such drugs, including themselves, thereby increasing the speed with which the drugs are eliminated. The drugs

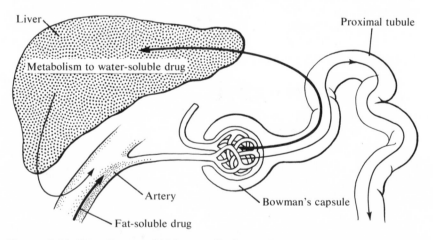

Figure 1.11. How liver and kidneys eliminate drugs from the body. Drugs may be filtered into the kidney, reabsorbed into the bloodstream, and carried to the liver for metabolic transformation to a more water-soluble compound that, having been filtered into the kidney, cannot be reabsorbed and is therefore excreted in urine.

induce an increase both in the enzyme activity of these cells and in the total amount of drug-metabolizing enzymes in the liver. Because these enzymes have a low specificity for drugs (that is, one enzyme may metabolize many different types of drugs), an increase in the metabolizing enzymes induced by one drug will increase the enzymes' rate of metabolizing that particular drug and a variety of others. This process will be elaborated upon later in this chapter, but it is important to note here that this enzyme-induction process is one mechanism for producing pharmacological *tolerance,* so that increasing doses of a drug must be administered in order to produce the same effect that smaller doses produced earlier.

Earlier, we discussed the processes of distribution of drugs from the mother to the fetus via the placenta. While the fetus is attached to the mother, drugs may be excreted through the umbilical cord back into the bloodstream of the mother. The mother can then eliminate the drug through the liver and kidneys. After delivery, however, the newborn baby is no longer attached to the mother and must get rid of the drug by itself. Unfortunately, the newborn (especially the premature infant) has few drug-metabolizing enzymes in the liver, and the kidneys may not yet be fully functional. Therefore, the infant has great difficulty metabolizing and excreting drugs. If it has received a high concentration of depressant drugs (anesthetics, narcotics, and so on) from the mother, the infant may be depressed for a long time after delivery.

Elimination of Drugs in Bile

Although excretion of drugs in bile is much less important than excretion by the kidney, many drugs, such as the antibiotics penicillin, streptomycin, and tetracycline, are excreted to a small extent in the bile. After one of these drugs has been metabolized by the liver, it is secreted by the liver cells into the bile and passes into the intestine. There, if it is fat soluble, it may be reabsorbed by the intestine into the bloodstream and excreted by the kidney. If it is highly water soluble, however, it will remain in the intestine and be excreted with the feces.

Elimination of Drugs by the Lungs

Certain drugs (including many anesthetics, nicotine from cigarettes, cannabinols from marijuana, and the narcotic agents in opium) may be absorbed through the lungs. Although they may be absorbed by this route, nicotine, cannabinols, and opiates are *not* excreted by the lungs. They are metabolized by the liver and excreted in the urine. Anesthetic gases, however, *are* excreted by the lungs. As soon as the anesthesiologist stops administering anesthetic to the patient, the concentration of the anesthetic in the lungs drops below the concentration of the anesthetic in the blood. Since these drugs are extremely fat soluble, they readily and rapidly pass back into the lungs from the bloodstream and are then exhaled in the patient's expired air, so that eventually anesthesia is terminated.

Elimination of Drugs in Body Secretions

Besides the kidneys, bile, and lungs, other possible routes for the excretion of drugs include sweat, saliva, and milk. Many drugs and drug metabolites may be found in these secretions, but their concentrations are usually quite low, and these routes are usually not considered to be among the primary paths of drug elimination. Occasionally, however, concern arises over the transfer of drugs (such as nicotine) from mothers to their breast-fed babies. Similarly, concern has been expressed about the secretion of antibiotics administered to cows into milk that is to be consumed by humans. These topics are of obvious importance to the pharmacologist and to the Food and Drug Administration, especially since guidelines for such uses of drugs must be drawn in order to minimize the possible danger to the public.

TOLERANCE AND DEPENDENCY

Drug *tolerance* may be defined as a state of progressively decreasing responsiveness to a drug. A person who develops tolerance requires a larger dose of the drug in order to achieve the effect originally obtained by a smaller dose.

Physical dependence is an entirely different phenomenon, even though it is associated with drug tolerance in most cases. A person physically dependent on a drug requires that drug in order to function normally. The state of physical dependence is revealed by withdrawing the drug and noting the occurrence of withdrawal symptoms (abstinence syndrome) some time after the drug is withheld. The symptoms of withdrawal can be terminated by readministration of the drug.

Tolerance and physical dependence are thought to occur in the central nervous system, at the level of the nerve cell. However, *indi-*

rect mechanisms may induce tolerance in the *absence* of physical dependence. For example, the administration of a barbiturate sedative may increase the amount of drug-metabolizing enzymes in the liver, with the result that some of the barbiturate would be metabolized faster and its sedative effect limited. Therefore, larger amounts of the drug will be needed to achieve an effect similar to that observed when the drug was administered for the first time if the tolerance is to be overcome.

A more specific example of this is presented in Table 1.1. In the experiment, rabbits were pretreated with three daily doses of pentobarbital (a short-acting barbiturate, to be discussed later). The rabbits were then given a single challenging dose of pentobarbital. The length of time that the rabbits slept and the amount of pentobarbital in the animals' bloodstreams at the time of awakening were measured and compared with the sleeping time and the blood levels of pentobarbital in rabbits that were not pretreated but that were given an identical dose of the drug. The data indicate that, although the pretreated animals slept less than half as long as the control rabbits, their blood levels of the drug upon awakening were approximately the same. Pretreatment had raised the animals' tolerance for the drug—not by affecting the "sleep center" in the brain, but by the induction of metabolizing enzymes in the liver that caused the drug to be metabolized and excreted more rapidly.

Such a mechanism of tolerance as the induction of drug-metabolizing enzymes does not, however, fully explain the tolerance and physical dependence that can develop with the use of many psychoactive drugs, for it accounts only for the necessity to double a

Table 1.1. Effect of Pentobarbital Pretreatment on the Duration of Pentobarbital Action. Rabbits were pretreated with three daily doses of pentobarbital (60 mg/kg) subcutaneously, then given a single challenging dose of 30 mg/kg intravenously.

Pretreatment	Sleeping time (minutes)	Plasma level of pentobarbital on awakening (μg/ml)	Pentobarbital half-life in plasma (minutes)
None	67 ± 4	9.9 ± 1.4	79 ± 3
Pentobarbital	30 ± 7	7.9 ± 0.6	26 ± 2

SOURCE: H. Remmer, "Drugs as Activators of Drug Enzymes," in *Metabolic Factors Controlling Duration of Drug Action* (Proceedings of First International Pharmacological Meeting), vol. 6, B. B. Brodie and E. G. Erdos, eds. (New York: Macmillan, 1962), p. 235.

dosage to produce a drug effect. It is not uncommon to see alcoholics and people dependent on sedatives to increase dosages by factors of 10 and others dependent on narcotic analgesics to increase dosages by factors of between 10 and 20. Therefore, there must exist (and there do exist) other mechanisms in the body that are responsible for the induction of tolerance and for the withdrawal state seen when certain drugs are removed. Such mechanisms appear to be situated within the brain but are as yet poorly identified.

DRUG SAFETY AND EFFECTIVENESS

We have discussed the general principles of how the body handles a drug, but before we discuss specific drugs, we should describe briefly several other factors that influence the effects of drugs on the body.

Obviously the rates of absorption, distribution, metabolism, and excretion to a large extent determine the intensity and duration of a drug's action. Other factors contributing to the drug response include (1) the possibility of one drug's affecting the body's response to another drug, (2) hypersensitivity to a drug, (3) allergy to a drug, and (4) individual sensitivity to a drug. Drug toxicity—both the side effects invariably associated with a drug and the more serious toxicities, including those that may be fatal—must always be considered.

Psychoactive drugs are usually classified according to their most prominent behavioral effect. Thus, drugs are classified as depressants, stimulants, hallucinogens, narcotics, and so on. However, for a true evaluation of a drug to be made, its effects should be related to the dosage administered.

The classification of a drug as a sedative does not adequately describe the actions of the compound, at least not until one understands all that the term *sedative* implies. (The implications are discussed in Chapter 3.) At low doses, a sedative may exert little or no effect; at moderate doses, the compound may induce sedation; at higher doses, it may put the patient to sleep; at extremely high doses, it may induce death. Thus, on the basis of dosage, this drug might be classified as a placebo (a compound that exerts no real effect), a sedative, a sleep-inducing agent, or a lethal substance.

The time course of drug action may be characterized by the latency of onset, the time taken to reach maximum effect, and the duration of the action. These characteristics are largely determined by the rates of absorption, distribution, metabolism, and excretion of the drug. A drug that is slowly absorbed will have a long latency of onset, whereas a drug administered intravenously may have an almost instantaneous onset of action. The time taken for the drug to reach peak effect is often determined by the distribution of the drug in the body. Those psychoactive drugs that cross the blood-brain barrier rapidly and reach nerve tissue quickly usually take a shorter time to reach maximum effect than do those drugs that only slowly gain access to the brain. For example, both thiopental (Pentothal) and pentobarbital (Nembutal) are sleep-inducing agents. Thiopental is more fat soluble than is pentobarbital and crosses the blood-brain barrier within an extremely short time (usually a few seconds). Pentobarbital, because it has some difficulty passing through the blood-brain barrier, may take many minutes to build up concentrations in the brain sufficient to induce sleep.

Similarly, rates of redistribution of a drug in the body, metabolism to inactive products, and excretion of the metabolized product determine the duration of drug action. Thiopental, with its high solubility in fat, rapidly leaves brain tissue and is carried to the muscles and fatty areas of the body. Thus, the blood levels of thiopental are quite low, so the patient awakens (the drug having left the brain, although not the body), and the drug is then slowly metabolized and excreted. Pentobarbital, being less soluble in fat, does not become redistributed to the fatty areas, so the blood levels of the drug are much higher, with the result that the patient is sedated for a prolonged time—until the drug is metabolized and excreted. In order for the sedative action of pentobarbital to be terminated, the drug must be metabolized by the liver and excreted in urine. As the dosage of the drug is increased, drug effects are usually perceived earlier and the duration of action is prolonged.

Drug Interactions

It is widely appreciated that the effects of one drug can be modified by the concurrent administration of another drug. For example, alcohol, taken after a sleeping pill or a "tranquilizer" (discussed in Chapter 3), will increase the loss of coordination and the sedation. This may be of little consequence if the dosages of each drug are low (one or two tablets and only one or two drinks), but higher dosages of either or both drugs can be dangerous both to the user and to others. If a person can normally ingest a limited amount of alcohol and still drive a car without significant loss of control or coordination, the concurrent ingestion of a tranquilizer may profoundly affect his or her driving performance, endangering driver, passengers, and other motorists. Literally hundreds of other examples could be given, and you should be aware of the danger in our society of significant interactions occurring when more than one drug is taken at the same time.

We have already discussed two of the prime factors contributing to drug interactions. First, many drugs are bound to plasma proteins and this binding serves as a reservoir of inactive drugs. If a second drug displaces a drug already bound to the protein (by competing for the same protein), more of the previously bound drug will be able to pass out of the bloodstream and be available to the receptor and thus a more intense effect may be produced: the displacing drug would increase the effects or the toxicity (or both) of the drug that was displaced.

Second, in our discussion of tolerance we stated that a drug that is metabolized by the liver may induce new enzymes, which can then metabolize any of a variety of other drugs. Thus, an enzyme-inducing drug such as pentobarbital (see Table 1.1) will decrease the activity of other drugs metabolized in the liver by increasing their rates of metabolism. Again, these illustrate the wide variety of factors influencing the magnitude of drug action in the body and point out that using more than one drug at any one time may be risky, whether the drugs are used separately or mixed in one concoction. Mixtures often complicate therapy since it often has not been established that more than one drug is needed, and if toxic effects should occur, it may be difficult to determine which drug is responsible.

Drug Toxicity

No drug is free of toxic effects, and while often they may be trivial, occasionally they are serious. As we mentioned earlier, no drug exerts a single effect; usually several different body functions are altered. These multiple effects of drugs occur despite the fact that one is usually interested in obtaining a single or perhaps a small number of the drug's many possible effects. The desired effect is usually considered to be the *main effect,* while the unwanted responses are labeled the *side effects.* To achieve the main effect, the side effects must be tolerated, which is possible if they are minor but may be limiting if they are more serious. The distinction between main and side effects is relative and depends on the purpose of the drug. What may be one person's side effect may be the main effect sought by another person. With morphine, for example, the pain-relieving properties may be sought, but the intestinal constipation induced is an undesired side effect and must be tolerated. However, morphine may also be used to treat diarrhea, so that the constipation induced is considered the main effect and any relief of pain a side effect.

Apart from irritating, but seldom dangerous, side effects, drugs occasionally induce more serious toxic manifestations, perhaps because of allergy or hypersensitivity to the drug. Serious blood disorders, toxicity to the liver or the kidney, or abnormal fetal development (teratogenesis) may be induced. The incidence of all of these serious toxic effects is fortunately quite low. Allergies to drugs may take many forms, from mild skin rashes to fatal shock caused by such drugs as penicillin. Allergy differs from normal side effects, which may often be eliminated, or at least made tolerable, by a simple reduction in the dose of the drug. A reduction in the dose may be *useless* for a drug allergy since exposure to *any* amount of the drug is hazardous and may be catastrophic.

Because drugs are concentrated, metabolized, and excreted by the liver and kidney, damage to these organs by drugs is not uncommon. An example of *drug-induced* liver damage is that caused by alcohol. Similarly, a class of major tranquilizers called the phenothiazines, of which chlorpromazine (Thorazine) is an example, may induce jaundice by increasing the viscosity of bile in the liver. Finally, infectious hepatitis may accompany drug injection if strict sterility is not observed.

The thalidomide tragedy dramatically illustrated that drugs may adversely influence fetal development. Much controversy has also arisen over the possible effects of LSD on fetal development. The seriousness of the problem of drug action on the fetus and the wide range of possible consequences was stated in one pharmacology textbook as follows:

> It is clear that the risks of chemical teratogenesis . . . are accentuated during the first trimester of pregnancy. Until much more information becomes available, the very diversity of known teratogens and mutagens (drugs that alter the structure of chromosomes in the cell) should dictate caution . . . A woman who is known to be pregnant should not be exposed to drugs at all during the first trimester unless the need is pressing. At least until experimental or statistical investigations show them to be harmless, caffeine, nicotine, and alcohol, to which people are so frequently exposed, should be regarded as possibly hazardous to the fetus during the first three months of pregnancy.[1]

The problem of teratogenesis, then, goes far beyond thalidomide and LSD and involves virtually every compound that is ingested or inhaled, including coffee, tea, cigarettes, and alcohol. More will be said about the toxicity of these agents in later chapters.

Placebo Effects

Pharmacology is concerned with the actions of drugs on biological mechanisms. The term *placebo,* however, refers to a pharmacologically *inert* substance that elicits a significant reaction. Since this action is independent of any chemical property of the drug (being inert), it arises largely because of what the individual expects, desires, or was told would happen. This placebo response seems to arise from a person's mental set or from the entire environmental situation or setting in which the drug is taken. In certain predisposed individuals, the placebo substance may produce extremely strong reactions with far-reaching consequences. The placebo effect may be particularly powerful and significant in the social use of alcohol and marijuana.

Even more remarkable is the demonstration that placebos may evoke patterns of altered behavior that have durations of action similar to those observed when a pharmacologically active drug is ingested. Thus, in discussing the pharmacology of a psychoactive agent, we must pay particular attention to the set, the setting, and the predisposition of the subjects if we are to describe the pharmacological effects of a drug accurately.

Responses closely mimicking those produced by pharmacologically active drugs can be learned in the complete absence of either drug or placebo. For instance, meditation techniques can produce states that closely resemble those produced by drugs, especially altered states of consciousness. It may, for example, be possible to use meditation to alter activity in certain centers of the brain in much the same way that a drug would alter the activity. Indeed, the placebo effect is a powerful element of drug-induced responses.

DEVELOPMENT OF NEW DRUGS

To complete our discussion of the effects of drugs in the body, let us describe briefly the processes and procedures through which new drugs are developed and evaluated before they are released for public use.

The earliest medicinal products were usually natural in origin: crude powders of leaves or roots, or extracts from a variety of plants or animals. One of the great advances of the twentieth century was the development of organic chemistry, which has made practical the synthesis of new drug molecules that, it is hoped, offer more promise than many products obtained from natural sources. Although new drugs are occasionally discovered by accident, they usually result from systematic and tedious laboratory investigation and careful scientific observation.

The development and marketing of new drugs in the United States is rigidly controlled by the federal government through the Food and Drug Administration (FDA). Before it is marketed for general clinical use, a new drug must be subjected to thorough laboratory and clinical pharmacological studies that demonstrate the usefulness and safety of the compound. Before studies in man are permitted, the pharmacology of a new drug must be extensively delineated in animals. These studies include the establishment of the range of effective doses, the doses at which side effects occur, and the lethal doses in various animals. The studies on the safety and toxicity of the drug are evaluated after administration of single doses and during long-term use. From all these studies, a risk/benefit ratio can be determined. Because of differences between species of animals, these studies must usually be carried out in at least three different species. In this preliminary testing on animals, neither the mechanism of the drug's action nor the range of its possible clinical usefulness need be completely described, although the absorption, distribution, metabolism, and excretion of the drug are carefully delineated.

Having been found safe to use in animals, the compound may be taken into initial clinical trial (phase 1), which is usually conducted on normal volunteer subjects, as well as on patients, and is aimed at establishing the drug's safety, dose range, and possible problems for further study. If phase 1 studies indicate safety, the drug may be subjected to a thorough clinical pharmacological evaluation (phase 2). These studies of necessity are closely controlled to eliminate such variables as placebo response and investigator bias. Statistical validation is of paramount importance. Finally, if a drug still looks promising, it will enter phase 3 of the human studies, a period of extended clinical evaluation. In this phase, the compound is made available to investigators throughout the country for use in a variety of clinical situations. This is done in order to elicit information about the drug's safety, efficacy, side effects, dosage, variability of response, and so on.

If a drug passes all of these trials, it may finally be approved by the FDA for sale to the public. However, most new drugs *never* get approval for marketing. Currently it is estimated to cost a pharmaceutical manufacturer approximately $9 million to take a new compound through laboratory and clinical testing to the stage of marketing. Although this attention to detail may seem almost excessive, it has been demonstrated to work to the benefit of the public. Most drugs currently on the legitimate market have reasonable risk/benefit ratios. No drug is completely without risk, but most drugs on the legitimate market are relatively safe.

NOTE

1. A. Goldstein, L. Aronow, and S. M. Kalman, *Principles of Drug Action* (New York: Harper & Row, 1968), p. 733.

Chapter 2

The Five Classes of Psychoactive Drugs: A Starting Point for Understanding

Some form of classification of psychoactive drugs into classes that lend themselves to coherent discussion is essential. There are at least three possible kinds of classification. Obviously, the best way would be according to the mechanism of action of each drug, but our knowledge of the physiology of the brain is too limited to organize drugs this way. A second method might be according to chemical structure, since, in some instances, drugs of similar chemical structure may be found to exert similar effects. However, too many drugs that appear to be similar in chemical structure are quite different in pharmacological activity. Conversely, drugs of quite different chemical structure may produce similar pharmacological actions. A third way would be to classify psychoactive drugs according to their legality or illegality, their potential for misuse, their potential hazards to health and public safety, and the like. However, these approaches are often based on current public opinion, laws, or emotion and are therefore frequently inconsistent with available pharmacological and medical information.

Table 2.1. Five Classes of Drugs that Alter Mood or Behavior. Only representative agents from each class of drug are listed. Brand names are shown in italics.

1. Sedative-Hypnotic Compounds (CNS Depressants)
   Barbiturates
     Long-acting: phenobarbital *(Luminal)*
     Intermediate-acting: amobarbital *(Amytal)*
     Short-acting: pentobarbital *(Nembutal)*, secobarbital *(Seconal)*
     Ultrashort-acting: pentothal *(Thiopental)*
   Nonbarbiturate hypnotics
     Glutethimide *(Doriden)*
     Methyprylon *(Noludar)*
     Methaqualone *(Parest, Quaalude, Somnafac, Sopor)*
   Antianxiety agents
     Meprobamate *(Miltown, Equanil)*
     Chlordiazepoxide *(Librium)*
     Diazepam *(Valium)*
   Others
     Ethyl alcohol; bromide; paraldehyde; chloral hydrate; anesthetic gases and
       liquids (ether, halothane, chloroform, etc.)

2. Behavioral Stimulants and Convulsants
   Amphetamines: *Benzedrine; Dexedrine; Methedrine*
   Clinical antidepressants
     Monoamine oxidase (MAO) inhibitors: *Parnate*
     Tricyclic compounds: *Tofranil; Elavil*
   Cocaine
   Convulsants: strychnine; *Metrazol; Picrotoxin*
   Caffeine
   Nicotine

3. Narcotic Analgesics (Opiates)
   Opium; heroin; morphine; codeine; *Numorphan; Dilaudid; Percodan; Demerol*

4. Antipsychotic Agents
   Phenothiazines: chlorpromazine *(Thorazine)*
   Reserpine *(Serpasil)*
   Butyrophenones: haloperidol *(Haldol)*
   Lithium

5. Psychedelics and Hallucinogens
   LSD (lysergic acid diethylamide)
   Mescaline
   Psilocybin
   Substituted amphetamines: DOM (STP); MDA; MMDA
   Tryptamine derivatives; DMT; DET; bufotenin
   Phencyclidine *(Sernyl)*
   Cannabis: marijuana; hashish; tetrahydrocannabinol

At present, the most realistic approach is to classify psychoactive drugs according to their most prominent behavioral effect or the effect that established their medical, behavioral, or recreational usefulness. Such a classification is presented in Table 2.1. The table lists five major classes of drugs that alter mood or behavior: the sedative-hypnotic compounds (depressants of the central nervous system), the behavioral stimulants and convulsants, the narcotic analgesics (the opiates), the antipsychotic agents (used in the treatment of psychoses), and, finally, a group of heterogeneous drugs referred to as the psychedelics and hallucinogens.

ASSUMPTIONS ABOUT THE CLASSIFICATION

There are five qualifications to be aware of as regards the usefulness of this table.

First, it should be noted that, in general, the action of psychoactive drugs is seldom restricted to any one functional or anatomical subdivision of the brain. There are exceptions, of course (such as the use of l-dopa for the treatment of Parkinson's disease), but usually a psychoactive drug will simultaneously affect a variety of processes. This complicates the classification of drugs since, at different doses of a drug, different behavioral actions may predominate. Some compromises must therefore be made.

Second, ultimately we may find that the action of any given psychoactive drug is explained by alterations in the synthesis, release, action, metabolism, and so on of a specific neurotransmitter chemical. (The neurochemical processes that mediate transmission of information between neurons are discussed at some length in Appendix II.) However, that neurotransmitter chemical may be involved in many different activities of the brain (norepinephrine, for example, may be involved in temperature regulation, arousal, satiety, rage, and so on). Thus, although a psychoactive drug might ultimately be found to exert a single effect on a specific neurotransmitter chemical, a variety of behavioral effects would be expected since this neurotransmitter is involved in many different functions.

Third, it is important to understand that psychoactive drugs do not create *new* behavioral or physiological responses; they simply *modify* ongoing processes. Current thought holds that the behavioral effects that psychoactive drugs exert are secondary to their blocking or modification of biochemical and/or physiological processes, particularly the various steps of synaptic transmission in the brain.

Fourth, the classification of psychoactive drugs in Table 2.1 is not rigid. Different behavioral responses are observed at different doses. Alcohol, for example, is classified as a general depressant compound, despite the fact that, at low doses, behavioral excitation may be observed. Thus, classification alone does not clearly describe the pharmacology of a drug. Classification, however, serves as a starting point from which several compounds may be compared and contrasted.

Finally, in the use of centrally acting drugs, certain factors that may lead to compulsive misuse of the drug must be considered. Such factors include physiological dependence, psychological dependence, and tolerance. Psychoactive drugs each differ in their potential to induce such hazards. It should be apparent, however, that any drug that is capable of favorably altering mood or behavior or of creating a pleasurable state of consciousness is capable of inducing psychological dependence—that is, a compulsion to use the drug for a favorable effect. This is not to state, however, that the use of a drug for recreation or to achieve pleasure is wrong.

THE FUTURE DISCUSSION

In subsequent chapters we will describe specific agents within each of the classes of psychoactive agents listed in the table. Alcohol and marijuana are discussed separately (in chapters 4 and 9). Both agents might well be included in the chapter on sedative-hypnotic compounds (Chapter 3), but because of their wide range of use, ready availability, and social and legal implications they deserve separate presentation.

Chapter 10 discusses the effects of body hormones on the brain and on behavior—for example, oral contraceptives and fertility agents. Although these are not directly related to psychoactive drugs, the chapter has been included because of the wide interest in such drugs. Since the limbic system, hypothalamus, and pituitary gland are thought to be important sites of action of these compounds, a discussion of their physiological, pharmacological, behavioral, and sociological effects seems pertinent.

Let us now consider the first category in the table: sedative-hypnotic compounds.

Chapter 3

Sedative-Hypnotic Compounds: Drugs that Depress the Central Nervous System

The sedative-hypnotic compounds are drugs of diverse chemical structure all capable of inducing varying degrees of behavioral depression. Such drugs are divided somewhat arbitrarily into (1) the barbiturates, (2) the nonbarbiturate hypnotics, (3) the antianxiety agents, and (4) a group of miscellaneous compounds not structurally related to those mentioned; alcohol, bromide, the general anesthetics, paraldehyde, and so on (see Table 2.1).

The classification of these compounds as sedative-hypnotics may be somewhat misleading. They are capable of inducing not only behavioral sedation or hypnosis (sleep) but also behavioral alterations, ranging from (at low doses) relief from anxiety, to sedation, release from inhibition, sleep, general anesthesia, coma, and finally (at high doses) death as a result of the depression of the respiratory

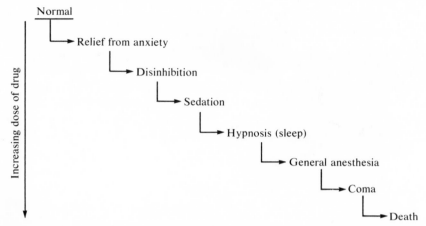

Figure 3.1. Continuum of behavioral sedation. How increasing doses of sedative-hypnotic drugs affect behavior.

centers in the medulla. (See Appendix II for a discussion of the anatomy of the brain.) This gradation of action is illustrated in Figure 3.1.

Virtually all of the sedative-hypnotic compounds discussed in this chapter are capable of inducing *any* of the states of behavioral depression depicted. Thus, depending upon the dose, any sedative-hypnotic compound may be classified as a *sedative,* a *tranquilizer,* a *hypnotic,* or an *anesthetic.* The compounds differ from one another, therefore, not in their sites of actions, uses, or abilities to induce various stages of depression, but in their individual potency and in the chemical differences that cause them to be handled differently by the body.

For example, a much smaller amount of secobarbital (a barbiturate) may be required to induce sleep than an amount of meprobamate (a dicarbamate) required to induce sleep. Therefore, secobarbital would be said to be more *potent.* But, comparison by potency is rather meaningless, since such factors as safety and efficacy may be more important in determining a compound's usefulness. (The dose-response relationship is discussed in Appendix V.)

FIVE PRINCIPLES OF CNS DEPRESSANTS

Since the sedative-hypnotic drugs are similar pharmacologically, let us discuss the barbiturates as a prototype class of agents and then compare other compounds with this prototype. Also, since all

CNS depressants are so similar in their actions, five general principles that apply fairly uniformly to all the CNS depressants can be summarized.

First, the effects of CNS depressants are *additive* with one another and with the behavioral state of the user. For example, alcohol will exaggerate the depression induced by barbiturates. Conversely, barbiturates will intensify the impairment of driving ability induced by alcohol. Similarly, a person who is depressed or physically tired may be profoundly affected by a dose of depressant drug that would only slightly affect a person who is behaviorally normal or excited.

Second, *antagonism* occurs between the CNS depressants and the behavioral stimulants. Such antagonism is usually nonspecific; that is, when a person is profoundly depressed by a sedative drug, the administration of a stimulant will seldom *specifically* block the action of that depressant and return the patient to normal, although the stimulant may temporarily arouse the patient. In fact, the stimulant may do more harm than good, because when it wears off, the patient will become even more depressed. What is needed clinically is a specific antagonist to CNS depressants, a drug that actually displaces the depressant from its receptors in the brain, thus immediately terminating the action of the depressant. Such a drug might save thousands of lives each year if it were used, for example, to treat individuals who had attempted suicide with CNS depressants (sleeping pills). Treatment of these individuals is at present difficult.

Third, current theory holds that general depressants exert a depressant action upon all neurons within the brain and, indeed, upon all tissues of the body. However, it is well known that low doses of these compounds induce behavioral excitement, a state that is often sought when a person wants to "get loaded" or "get drunk." The excitement is thought to be due to a depression of inhibitory neurons within the brain, which leaves one in a state of *disinhibition*. Because alcohol often induces euphoria, one frequently finds alcohol classified mistakenly as a stimulant rather than as a depressant. It is believed that, at low doses of alcohol (or other depressant), inhibitory synapses in the brain are depressed slightly earlier than are excitatory synapses. If inhibition is depressed, behavioral excitation would be observed, since all neurons within the brain are held in a close balance between excitation and inhibition, and this would appear to account for the euphoria induced by low doses of sedative-hypnotic drugs. At higher doses, however, excitatory synapses also are depressed and sleep follows.

Methaqualone (the "love drug," see below) provides another example of the misclassification of a depressant drug. Methaqualone is a sedative-hypnotic agent of moderately low potency that, like all depressant drugs, is capable of inducing a state of disinhibition or euphoria at certain doses. During such disinhibition one might certainly feel more euphoric about sexual experiences, but such feelings are limited by at least two factors: (1) while sensation may be increased, performance may be decreased, and (2) since the effect depends on the dose, overdoses induce sleep or (with higher doses) deeper levels of behavioral depression.

Fourth, in general, behavioral depression induced by a single dose of depressant drug is seldom followed by a period of either mental or behavioral hyperexcitability after the drug action is terminated. As the drug is metabolized and excreted, the individual slowly reverts from a depressed state to a normal one. However, if large doses of depressants are *repeatedly* administered over a prolonged period of time, the depression induced *is* followed by a period of hyperexcitability which, upon withdrawal of the drug, may be quite severe and might even lead to convulsions and death. These agents, therefore, are capable of inducing physiological dependency.

Fifth, use of the sedative-hypnotic compounds has the inherent capability of inducing psychological dependence and tolerance as well: tolerance secondary both to the induction of drug-metabolizing enzymes in the liver (so that the drug is metabolized more rapidly) and to the adaptation of cells in the brain so that they will function in the presence of the drug—neurons become tolerant of the presence of the drug and larger doses must then be administered in order to obtain a given behavioral effect.

In addition, a remarkable degree of *cross tolerance* may occur. This is a condition in which tolerance to one drug results in a lessened response to another drug. *Cross dependence,* too, may be exhibited. This is a condition in which one drug can prevent withdrawal symptoms associated with physical dependence on a different drug. Essentially, any sedative-hypnotic drug can substitute for any other in the same class, regardless of chemical structure.

HISTORICAL BACKGROUND

The use of depressant compounds is as old as history. Alcohol is the oldest of the depressant agents and in earlier days was held to be a remedy for practically all diseases and problems. In fact, in the

Middle Ages alcohol was believed to be the long-sought elixir of life. More recent history of depressant drugs began with the discovery of nitrous oxide (laughing gas) by Joseph Priestley in 1772. However, nitrous oxide did not become widely used in medicine as an anesthetic for approximately 100 years and was then soon followed by other anesthetic agents, including ether and chloroform.

Although barbituric acid was first prepared in 1864, it was not until 1903 that the first barbiturate derivative was introduced into medicine as a sedative drug. This was followed in 1912 by the commercial introduction of phenobarbital. Since that time, more than 2,500 barbiturates have been synthesized and approximately 50 have been marketed.

These agents (together with other depressant compounds such as bromide and paraldehyde) were the only available general depressants until the early 1950s when meprobamate was introduced as a "minor tranquilizer." (In reality, meprobamate appears to be pharmacologically very similar to the barbiturates introduced many years earlier, and the term "minor tranquilizer" is more a sales gimmick than a pharmacological description.) Then in about 1960, chlordiazepoxide (Librium) became the first available benzodiazepine tranquilizer. This compound and its derivative, diazepam (Valium), share many of the characteristics of the general depressant agents and thus are presented in this chapter as general CNS depressants. Although there are recent claims that the benzodiazepines may have some separate, more specific actions in the limbic system, where a calming of aggressive behavior may be induced at doses that do not seem to induce behavioral depression, at slightly higher doses the benzodiazepines appear to resemble the other CNS depressants closely.

SITE AND MECHANISM OF ACTION

The barbiturates and other sedative-hypnotic compounds are general depressants. That is, they depress the activity of the brain, the nerves, the muscles, and the heart tissue, they reduce the rate of metabolism in a variety of tissues throughout the body, and, in general, they depress any system that uses energy. Most of these depressant effects, however, require high concentrations of drug. In *normal doses,* the sedative-hypnotic compounds appear to be selective depressants of certain pathways within the brain that are involved in wakefulness. More specifically, the behavioral-depressant action of these compounds appears to result from an action on the arousal centers within the brain: the ascending reticular activating system (the ARAS), in the reticular formation, and the diffuse thalamic projection system. As we shall discuss in Chapter 5, these two centers within the brainstem and midbrain are important for the maintenance of behavioral arousal.

Depression of synaptic transmission processes within these centers appears to account for the various stages of behavioral depression induced by the sedative-hypnotic drugs. Indeed, the processes of synaptic transmission are much more sensitive to these drugs than is the process of conduction along axons. Since these compounds depress synaptic transmission, one would expect that pathways that have many synapses would be especially susceptible to drug-induced depression. Indeed, physiological studies have demonstrated that the ARAS and the diffuse thalamic projection system are composed of multitudes of such polysynaptic pathways, which would account for the unusual sensitivity of these areas to depressant drugs.

DRUG-INDUCED "BRAIN SYNDROME"

In certain psychiatric and neurological disorders, such as the dementias, a behavioral pattern characteristic of depressed nerve function is observed. To diagnose this and other psychiatric disorders, a mental status examination is performed by the physician. This examination encompasses 12 areas of mental function, as listed in Table 3.1.

Table 3.1. The Mental Status Examination. Twelve areas of mental function.

 1. General appearance
 2. Sensorium:
      a. orientation to time, place, and person
      b. clear vs. clouded
 3. Behavior and mannerisms
 4. Stream of talk
 5. Cooperativeness
 6. Mood: inner feelings
 7. Affect: surface expression of feelings
 8. Perception:
      a. illusions: misperception of reality
      b. hallucinations: not present in reality
 9. Thought processes: logical vs. strange or bizarre
10. Mental content: fund of knowledge
11. Intellectual functions: ability to reason and interpret
12. Insight and judgment

Different psychiatric disorders manifest themselves as differing deficits in this examination. Schizophrenics, for example, have an intact sensorium, adequate memory, cooperativeness and behavior, and may speak with a normal stream of talk. Their mental status examination is characterized by disturbed thought processes with absence of logic and, frequently, with misperceptions of reality. (The pathological processes possibly involved in schizophrenia are further discussed in Chapter 7.)

In instances where neurons are reversibly depressed (as in intoxication with alcohol or other sedative-hypnotic drugs) or irreversibly damaged (as in dementia), five of the functions of the mental status examination are particularly altered: sensorium, affect, mental content, intellectual function, and insight and judgment. For example, when a person is intoxicated with alcohol or barbiturates, sensorium is clouded (rather than clear) and the individual is disoriented as to time and place. Memory is impaired and there is frequently a retrograde amnesia with loss of short-term (recent) memory. The intellect is depressed and judgment is decreased. The individual's affect is shallow and labile; that is, he is very vulnerable to external stimuli and may be sullen and moody at one moment and exhibit a mock anger at the next. When such a mental status is seen, it is diagnosed as a "brain syndrome" secondary to depressed nerve-cell function.

Of interest in the brain syndrome induced by sedative-hypnotic drugs is that certain individuals (such as the elderly) who already have some natural loss of nerve-cell function are more likely to be adversely affected by these drugs. A person whose sensorium is partially clouded or who is somewhat disoriented may become even more so when these drugs are taken. The net result is increased disorientation and further clouding of consciousness. Frequently, this is manifested as a state of drug-induced "paradoxical excitement," characterized by a labile personality with marked anger, delusions, hallucinations, and confabulations. The treatment of such a drug-induced disorder is discontinuation of the sedative drug.

THE BARBITURATES

The term *barbiturate* refers to those chemical compounds that are derivatives of barbituric acid (Figure 3.2). The barbiturates are capable of producing all degrees of behavioral depression, ranging from mild sedation, through anesthesia, to coma and death. The

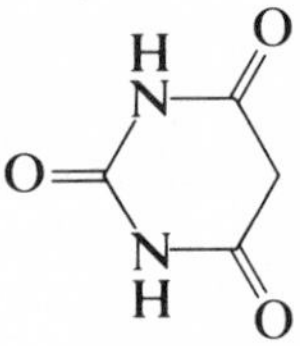

Barbituric acid 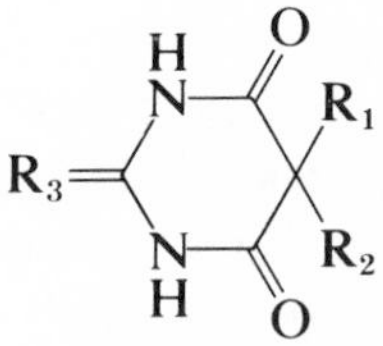   Barbiturate nucleus

Drug	R_1	R_2	R_3	Duration of action
Pentobarbital (Nembutal)	$-C_2H_5$	$-C_5H_{11}$	O =	Short
Secobarbital (Seconal)	$-CH_2-CH=CH_2$	$-C_5H_{11}$	O =	Short
Amobarbital (Amytal)	$-C_2H_5$	$-C_5H_{11}$	O =	Intermediate
Phenobarbital (Luminal)	$-C_2H_5$	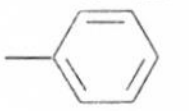 ⬡	O =	Long
Thiopental (Pentothal)	$-C_2H_5$	$-C_5H_{11}$	S =	Ultrashort

Figure 3.2. Chemical formulas of commonly used barbiturates. The symbols R_1, R_2, and R_3 on the barbiturate nucleus show the positions of the side groups that distinguish these compounds, and the side groups for each compound are listed in the table.

extent of the drug effect depends on several factors: the particular agent in question, the dose, the route of administration, the behavioral state of the individual when the drug is administered, and the rates of absorption, distribution, metabolism, and excretion. Thus, to describe the pharmacology of the barbiturates, we should distinguish the effects observed with the various types over a wide range of doses. Furthermore, the handling of the various types by the body should be compared and contrasted to determine the onset, intensity, and duration of the drug effect. Finally, the context in which barbiturates are taken must be carefully identified and evaluated in order to determine the effect of set and setting on the response.

Absorption, Distribution, Metabolism, and Excretion

As shown in Table 2.1 in Chapter 2, the barbiturates are subclassified into compounds of *ultrashort-, short-, intermediate-,* and *long-acting* durations of action. The placement of any given drug within one of these subclasses is determined by the rates of absorption, distribution, metabolism, and excretion of the compound.

For example, barbiturates in the stomach are in a fat-soluble form. Because of this they are rapidly and completely absorbed from stomach and upper intestine into the bloodstream; therefore, they are usually administered by mouth. Occasionally, however, an ultrashort-acting barbiturate is administered intravenously for use as a general anesthetic. This is a difficult technique and intravenous administration of barbiturates is usually not attempted except in emergencies or when adequate provisions are made for supporting respiration and circulation (and therefore life) in case of untoward reaction. Fatal accidents have resulted from the intravenous administration of barbiturates by inexperienced persons.

The barbiturates are well distributed to most of the tissues of the body. The ultrashort-acting compounds are very soluble in fat and therefore penetrate the blood-brain barrier easily and rapidly. These compounds, therefore, induce sleep within an extremely short period of time (usually within seconds). The long-acting barbiturates, by contrast, exist in blood in a more water-soluble form, which penetrates the blood-brain barrier with slightly more difficulty. Thus, induction of sleep with the long-acting compounds is delayed. The short-acting and intermediate-acting barbiturates are intermediate in fat solubility between the long-acting compounds and the ultrashort-acting compounds. They penetrate the brain within a period of several minutes after absorption.

The duration of barbiturate action in the body is determined by metabolism and excretion. Within a few minutes after an ultrashort-acting barbiturate (thiopental, for example) is administered, the drug rapidly leaves the brain (so its action is cut short) and is *redistributed* to other tissues, primarily the muscles and fat deposits such as adipose tissue. The ultrashort-acting barbiturates are then slowly metabolized by the liver and excreted by the kidneys, which is why people who have been sedated or anesthetized with thiopental may, even though they awaken within a very few minutes, find that they are groggy for several hours afterward. This grogginess is the result of the low levels of the drug that are being maintained in the blood while it is being slowly metabolized and excreted. The drug is still present; it is only that the concentration in the brain is not high enough to induce sleep or anesthesia.

The long-acting barbiturates (such compounds as phenobarbital) exist in the blood primarily in a water-soluble form and to a lesser extent in a fat-soluble form. Therefore, these compounds are only slightly soluble in muscle and body fat and they circulate in the bloodstream in concentrations sufficient to keep the individual sedated or drowsy until such time as the drug is either metabolized by the liver or excreted by the kidneys. This persistence of significant amounts of drug in the bloodstream to a large extent accounts for the hangover that lasts for several hours or even days after one of these agents has been ingested.

Thus, in summary, three processes are responsible for the termination of the depressant action of the barbiturates: *redistribution* to the muscle and fat, *metabolism* by the liver, and *excretion* by the kidneys. The process of redistribution is of primary importance in the termination of the hypnosis induced by the ultrashort-acting barbiturates, while excretion of drug by the kidneys (usually following metabolism of the drug by the liver) is essential for the termination of the hypnotic action of the long-acting compounds.

Uses

All of the barbiturates may be used for one or more of the reasons listed in Table 3.2. Most of these uses are based on the ability of the drugs to produce sedation or sleep, or to prevent epileptic seizures. The *primary* use of the barbiturates is to produce a state of drowsiness or sedation. The various barbiturates are widely prescribed whenever general behavioral depression is desired. Indeed, the barbiturates (especially those with long durations of action) are widely used as daytime sedatives (tranquilizers). Relief from anxiety and a state of euphoria frequently accompany the tranquility obtained from low doses of barbiturates or a combination of a barbiturate with another depressant drug such as alcohol. In higher doses, the barbiturates are useful to induce sleep, as general anesthetics for surgery, and to prevent convulsions.

There are several limitations to the use of barbiturates. These compounds are *not* analgesic and therefore they are *not* used for the relief of pain. In addition, the depressant action of these compounds upon the brainstem can interfere seriously with respiration (to the extent of causing death), especially when used intravenously or in suicide attempts. The other problems associated with these compounds (dependency, tolerance, and loss of coordination) will be discussed below.

Table 3.2. Major Uses of Sedative-Hypnotic Drugs

---

1. Medical
      Induction of sleep
      Daytime sedation
      Treatment of epileptic seizures
      Induction of anesthesia (ultrashort-acting compounds)
      Preanesthetic medication before surgery
      Treatment of anxiety and neuroses

2. Social and Recreational
      Relief from anxiety
      Induction of disinhibition or euphoria

Pharmacological Effects

At normal doses, the general depressant action of barbiturates is largely restricted to synapses in the CNS. The initial brain-wave alterations induced by the barbiturates are toward a high-voltage, low-frequency pattern characteristic of slow-wave sleep.

Normal sleep (not drug-induced) is a complex physiological process involving alternating episodes of rapid-eye-movement (REM) sleep and slow-wave sleep. Since barbiturate-induced sleep is characterized by slow waves, REM sleep is absent. Since dreaming occurs during REM sleep and is largely absent during slow-wave sleep, barbiturate-induced sleep differs from normal sleep in that the time spent in REM sleep is greatly reduced and dreaming is suppressed. In fact, some investigators think that this absence of REM sleep with loss of dreaming may be harmful and may even be capable of precipitating psychotic episodes. Individuals on barbiturates and deprived of REM sleep exhibit an increase in the proportion of time spent in REM sleep after they have stopped taking the drug—one example of a withdrawal effect following prolonged periods of barbiturate-induced depression.

Symptoms of drowsiness or a hangover may follow the use of a barbiturate. Such drowsiness, resulting from the presence of the drug in the body, may last for only a few hours, but more subtle alterations of judgment, motor skills, and behavior may persist for hours or days until the compound is removed from the body. Such a hangover closely resembles that following intoxication by alcohol.

Other physiological effects of the barbiturates are relatively minor, except for the depressant effects on respiration, which are minimal at sedative doses but result in death when an overdose is taken. The barbiturates appear to have no significant effects on the cardiovascular system, the gastrointestinal tract, the kidneys, or other organs until toxic doses are reached. In the liver, however, barbiturates stimulate the synthesis of enzymes that metabolize barbiturates and some other drugs, an effect that produces a degree of tolerance to such drugs.

Psychological Effects

Many of the behavioral effects of the barbiturates are quite similar to those observed during alcohol-induced inebriation and may even be indistinguishable from them. Barbiturates may initially produce behavioral disinhibition, presumably by depressing the central inhibitory synapses. This disinhibition (coupled with the relief from anxiety that is produced by small amounts of sedation) may result in a mild state of euphoria. Occasionally, however, as with alcohol, an individual may react by withdrawing, becoming emotionally depressed, or becoming aggressive and violent. Higher doses (or low doses combined with a dose of another depressant drug) lead to behavioral depression and sleep.

The individual's mental set and the physical or social setting in which the drug is ingested are important because they may largely determine whether a person experiences relief from anxiety or exhibits mental depression, aggression, or other unexpected or unpredictable responses.

An additional behavioral effect of consequence is the ataxia (staggering) and loss of motor coordination that may accompany use of depressant drugs. For instance, driving skills will be severely impaired by barbiturates and should be considered as a predictable consequence of the use of these drugs. The effects of barbiturates are additive with the effects produced by any other depressant compound (including alcohol) that may be in the blood. Thus, the behavior of one who normally can tolerate a given dose of a barbiturate might be noticeably affected if alcohol or another depressant were present in the bloodstream. Such additive effects might be of little consequence if low doses of both drugs were ingested, but they might lead to more serious consequences if one attempted to drive an automobile, for example. When relatively high doses of barbiturates are combined with relatively large amounts of alcohol, profound depression is induced and numerous accidental overdoses, leading to respiratory failure and death, have resulted from such combinations.

Adverse Reactions

SIDE EFFECTS AND TOXICITY

One of the primary effects induced by the use of barbiturates is drowsiness. Obviously, such drowsiness is often the main effect a person seeks. Quite frequently, however, when one is seeking a state of disinhibition or relief from anxiety, drowsiness is a necessary side effect.

Another side effect is impaired performance and judgment. As one text puts it:

> A person need not be rendered staggering drunk before his motor performance and, probably more important, his judgment are significantly impaired. The most common offending agent in this regard

is alcohol. . . . At this time it should be emphasized that all sedatives are equivalent to alcohol in their effects; that all are additive in their effects with alcohol; and that their effects persist longer than might be predicted.[1]

Other side effects are usually minor and include such actions as slight decreases in blood pressure and heart rate (as occur during natural sleep), drug-induced hangover, and other effects on various systems of the body that are not significant enough to merit discussion here.

TOLERANCE

The barbiturates are capable of inducing at least two types of tolerance: (1) that following the induction of metabolizing enzymes in the liver, and (2) that following the adaptation of neurons in the brain to the presence of the drug. As we discussed in Chapter 1, many barbiturates are capable of inducing enzymes in the liver that metabolize the barbiturates and many other drugs that might be in the body at that time. Thus, subsequently, a higher dose would be required to maintain a given level of drug in the body. In other words, more drug would have to be given in order to achieve the same concentration of drug at the receptor and thus achieve the same effect—assuming that the receptor did not become insensitive to the drug.

That assumption, however, is not necessarily true. It appears that receptors within the brain are capable of adapting to the presence of barbiturates. Therefore, more drug would have to be presented to the receptor in order to stimulate it to the same level. Therefore, the doses would have to be larger for two reasons: first, to maintain an adequate amount of the drug in the blood and, second, to raise the blood levels in order to stimulate the receptor to the same extent.

An individual does not necessarily develop tolerance to *all* the effects of the barbiturates. The tolerance we have described is primarily restricted to the sedative effects. The respiratory centers in the brainstem apparently *do not* become tolerant of the presence of barbiturates. As you will recall from the discussion of safety in Chapter 1, a risk/benefit ratio must be calculated for the drug. If the patient tolerates the drug-induced euphoria and behavioral sedation but not the respiratory-depressant effects of the drugs, the risks associated with the use of the drug would progressively *increase* as that tolerance develops; in essence, the margin of safety in the use of the drug would decrease. Thus, since the concentration of drug in the blood that will produce respiratory failure remains approximately the same for an individual, the person using increasingly larger doses of barbiturates for social or recreational purposes risks taking a dose that may be severely toxic or even lethal.

PHYSICAL DEPENDENCE

Barbiturates induce physical dependence. Withdrawal symptoms appear when administration of the drug is stopped. Physical dependence on the barbiturates is in some respects similar to the physical dependence induced by the opiate narcotics (see Chapter 6), but differs in two important respects. First, the dose of barbiturate required to induce physical dependence is much higher than the dose usually required to induce sleep. For example, approximately 100 milligrams of pentobarbital (Nembutal) will induce sleep, and serious physical dependence does not develop until, as tolerance builds, the patient reaches daily doses of 800 milligrams or more. Also it is usually only after such large doses of drug are reached that removal of the drug leads to *serious* and possibly lethal withdrawal symptoms. Opiate withdrawal may produce severe symptoms when even *normal* doses are discontinued. This is not to say, however, that normal doses of barbiturates may not produce some degree of physical dependence and symptoms of withdrawal when discontinued, but such symptoms at low doses are not usually serious or life threatening. Among the symptoms is a rebound increase in REM sleep. Patients experiencing this rebound may find it difficult to sleep and may be quite irritable for days or weeks after the barbiturate is discontinued.

Second, barbiturate withdrawal also differs from opiate withdrawal in that the former may lead to convulsions sometimes so serious as to be life threatening. Withdrawal from the opiate narcotics, however, is not usually as dangerous. Associated with these barbiturate-induced withdrawal convulsions may be periods of hallucination, restlessness, disorientation, and so on. Such withdrawal hyperexcitability is even more serious in an epileptic patient, who is more prone to severe convulsions. In such patients, serious withdrawal convulsions may be observed even when rather low doses of barbiturates are discontinued.

PSYCHOLOGICAL DEPENDENCE

Psychological dependence refers to a compulsion to use a drug for a pleasurable effect. All sedative-hypnotics are apt to be abused compulsively, the most abused being alcohol. The sedative-hypnotics together form one of our most widely used classes of psychoactive drugs. Each year we ingest enough barbiturates such that if every-body were to consume his or her yearly allotted dose at one time, we would kill the entire population from respiratory depression three times over. Indeed, approximately 3,000 deaths a year occur from overdoses. Use of barbiturates to this extent suggests that psychological dependence occurs in many individuals. Since they are capable of relieving anxiety, inducing sedation, and producing a state of euphoria, these drugs may be used to achieve a variety of psychological states. Many individuals in our society (especially older people) appear to be psychologically dependent upon the hypnotic effect of the barbiturates.

NONBARBITURATE HYPNOTICS

At approximately the same time that meprobamate was introduced into medicine, the nonbarbiturate sedatives, glutethimide (Doriden) and methyprylon (Noludar), were introduced as new drugs that produced sedation and sleep. In reality these are not strictly new drugs, since their structures are virtually identical with the barbiturates except for one slight modification of the molecule (see Figure 3.3). The pharmaceutical industry frequently makes minor changes in a basic chemical molecule and comes up with a "new" compound that may be patented and released for sale to obtain some of the sales enjoyed by the original product. Many of these compounds are still

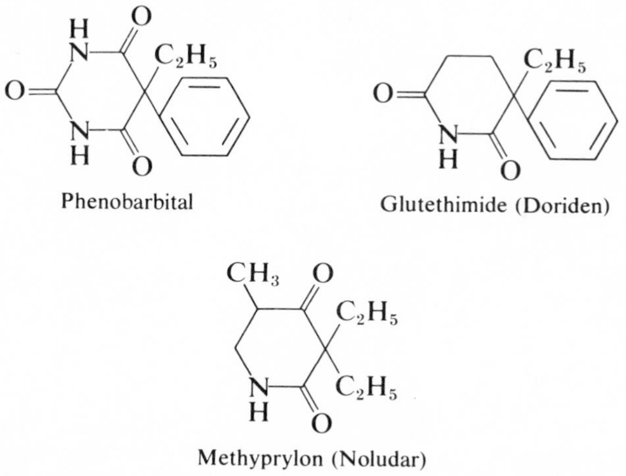

Phenobarbital

Glutethimide (Doriden)

Methyprylon (Noludar)

Figure 3.3. Structural formulas of phenobarbital (a barbiturate) and two nonbarbiturate hypnotics. Note the close structural resemblance of the nonbarbiturate compounds to phenobarbital.

similar to the original and produce identical effects. We mention nonbarbiturate hypnotics here, not to confuse the reader unduly, but to demonstrate that what is sold as a "nonbarbiturate" is in reality so close to the barbiturates that the receptors in the brain upon which barbiturates act probably cannot differentiate between them. Yet these nonbarbiturates may be promoted by drug companies as something "new."

MEPROBAMATE

Meprobamate (Miltown, Equanil), a sedative-hypnotic, is only one of a large number of dicarbamate derivates currently on the market and available on prescription (see Figure 3.4). Meprobamate and related dicarbamates are frequently referred to as minor tranquilizers or antianxiety agents. Frequently they are simply referred to as tranquilizers. The term tranquilizer, however, is misleading, as the true tranquilizers (the *major* tranquilizers) are the antipsychotic agents used in the treatment of psychosis and psychotic states (see Chapter 7). Meprobamate was one of the first tranquilizers to be introduced into the United States. Physicians began using it in the early 1950s as an alternative sedative-hypnotic product to alcohol and the barbiturates. Somehow the use of the term *tranquilizer* to describe meprobamate served to distinguish the product from the bar-

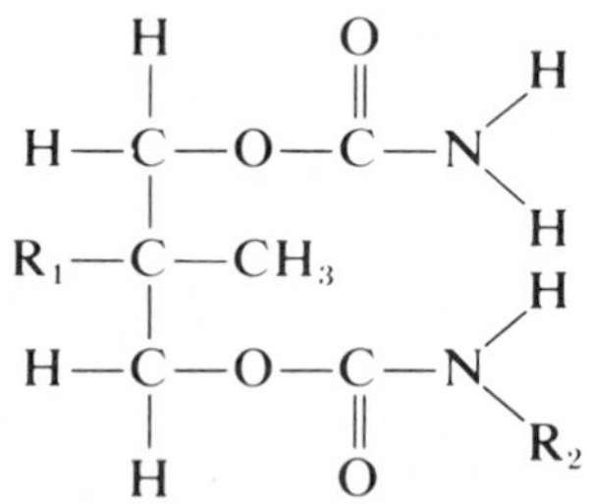

Dicarbamate nucleus

Drug	R_1	R_2
Meprobamate (Equanil, Miltown)	H_7C_3-	$-H$
Mebutamate (Capla)	H_9C_4-	$-H$
Carisoprodol (Rela, Soma)	H_7C_3-	$-C_3H_7$
Tybamate (Solacen, Tybatran)	H_7C_3-	$-C_4H_9$

Figure 3.4. Chemical formulas of meprobamate and other dicarbamate sedatives. The positions of the side groups listed in the table are indicated by R_1 and R_2 on the dicarbamate nucleus.

biturates, a distinction that now appears to be more theoretical than real. Low doses of barbiturates are effective as daytime sedatives and as antianxiety agents, while higher doses induce sleep. The same appears to be true for meprobamate. Doses of between 200 and 400 milligrams produce long-lasting daytime sedation, euphoria, and relief from anxiety; higher doses induce sleep.

Meprobamate is well absorbed orally and is usually not administered by injection. It is rapidly distributed to the brain and, since it is readily reabsorbed from the kidney, it must be metabolized before excretion. Therefore, meprobamate has a long duration of action and the sedation it induces will last for 10 hours or longer.

In general, meprobamate and the barbiturates induce the same pharmacological and toxicological effects. Tolerance, physical dependence, and psychological dependence can be induced to approximately the same extent with meprobamate and the barbiturates. Withdrawal symptoms when chronic administration of high doses of meprobamate is abruptly stopped may include convulsions, coma, psychotic behavior, and even death. It is somewhat more difficult, however, to commit suicide with meprobamate than with the barbiturates because meprobamate is not as potent a respiratory depressant as the barbiturates are and thus its margin of safety is greater. Successful suicide following the ingestion of meprobamate is rare, probably owing to this rather low potency.

BENZODIAZEPINES

Through the 1950s, the only sedative-hypnotic agents available were alcohol, the barbiturates, meprobamate, and the nonbarbiturate derivatives, glutethimide and methyprylon. In 1960, the first benzodiazepine, chlordiazepoxide (Librium), was introduced. To date, five additional benzodiazepines have been marketed and several others are awaiting introduction. The compounds include diazepam (Valium), oxazepam (Serax), flurazepam (Dalmane), clonazepam (Clonopin), and chlorazepate (Tranxene).

As can be seen from the chemical formulas (compare Figure 3.5 with Figure 3.2) the benzodiazepines are structurally unrelated to the barbiturates, but, pharmacologically, they closely resemble them. In fact, since the introduction of chlordiazepoxide in 1960, there has been controversy about the superiority of the benzodiazepines over the sedative-hypnotic compounds, including the barbiturates. Today, however, it is becoming increasingly clear that the benzodiazepines

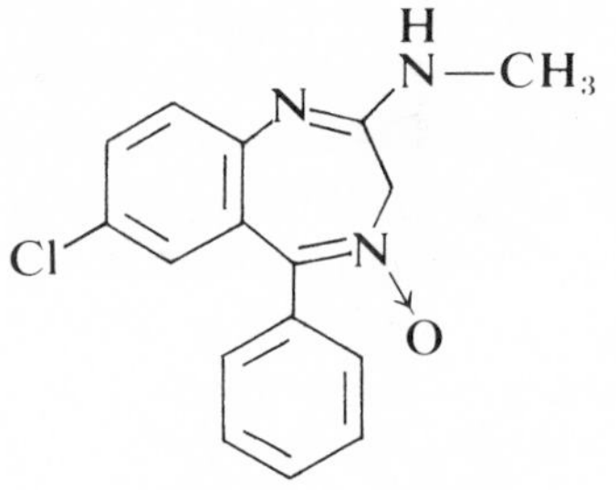

Chlordiazepoxide (Librium) 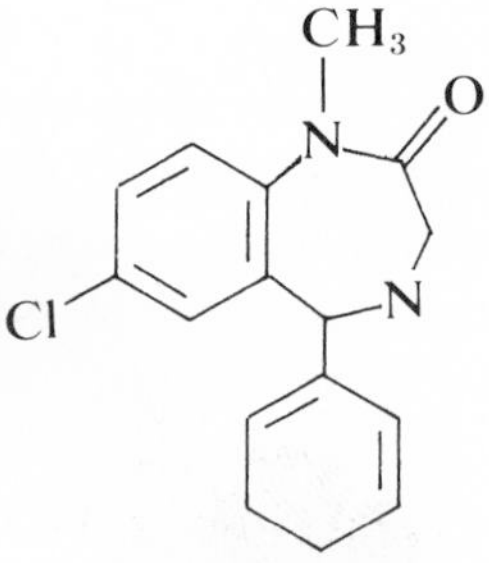   Diazepam (Valium)

Figure 3.5. Structural formulas of two benzodiazepine tranquilizers.

are somewhat more selective than the barbiturates in suppressing anxiety. More certain is the fact that the benzodiazepines are less hypnotic (sleep producing), although they are just as effective as sedatives. In addition, while barbiturates profoundly depress respiration in overdosage, it is extremely difficult to commit suicide by an overdose of a benzodiazepine. While these agents may cause some respiratory depression in high doses, such depression is seldom severe and rarely, if ever, fatal.

The wide acceptance of these compounds within our society is indicated by the fact that diazepam and chlordiazepoxide are currently the two most widely prescribed drugs in the United States. More than 65 million prescriptions for diazepam are filled each year. Only slightly less than this number are filled for chlordiazepoxide. Such use also leads to extensive misuse. In a recent federal government Drug Abuse Warning Network report, diazepam was listed as the "number one" drug seen for visits to emergency rooms across the nation. It was listed as the first or second most abused drug by 19 of the 23 reporting cities, and it was mentioned in more than 27,000 episodes of drug abuse. Seventy percent of these episodes involved women, and suicide attempts were involved in 51 percent of all incidents.

The benzodiazepines are only incompletely absorbed when taken orally, probably because they are in a water-soluble form in the stomach and thus are not absorbed to any significant extent until they reach the intestine. As a result, absorption is slow; it often takes between 8 and 24 hours to reach maximum levels in the bloodstream. Distribution to the brain is also slow, and levels of these drugs are maintained in the blood for several days, giving them a long duration of action.

Clinically, the benzodiazepines are used primarily for the treatment of anxiety, tension, behavioral excitement, and insomnia. They are also used as muscle relaxants, although the therapeutic effect here is debatable. Administration is almost universally oral. The only intravenous use is in the emergency treatment of severe epileptic convulsions.

As mentioned, six benzodiazepines are currently available. All have similar actions and they differ from each other principally in the methods through which they are promoted. For example, flurazepam (Dalmane) is promoted primarily as a hypnotic (sleep-inducing) compound. Clonazepam (Clonopin) is marketed for use in epilepsy. The other four benzodiazepines are promoted primarily as antianxiety drugs. In fact, two of these agents (diazepam and chlorazepate) are metabolized to oxazepam (Serax), which appears to be the "active" agent for all three. All three drugs, therefore, are essentially identical.

Their pharmacological similarity to the barbiturates and the other sedative-hypnotic compounds makes it seem likely that the benzodiazepines would induce tolerance and dependence. Indeed, some degree of tolerance can be measured after repeated administration but does not appear to be as marked as that induced by the barbiturates. Similarly, physical dependence, evidenced by withdrawal signs like those observed when barbiturates and other sedative agents are withdrawn, has been described. Finally, since these agents may produce relaxation and induce behavioral disinhibition, a feeling of well-being, and euphoria (all of which are similar to the effects induced by the barbiturates or alcohol), some degree of psychological dependence would be expected. Excessive use of the benzodiazepines may produce undesirable behavior, including disorientation, confusion, rage, and other symptoms resembling those of drunkenness. When used in the elderly or others with some loss of nerve-cell function (as we discussed earlier), these agents will further cloud the sensorium and will impair judgment and memory, resulting in a state of excitement, disorientation, and delirium. Treatment consists of stopping the medication.

Since these compounds are sedative agents, their effects are additive with those of other sedative-hypnotic compounds. Thus, while a clinical dose of a benzodiazepine may not severely impair driving performance, the addition of alcohol may induce significant impairment—probably one of the greatest impediments to the social use of these agents. At the moment, although we seriously try to prevent individuals from driving while under the influence of alcohol, we are not yet serious about restraining individuals who ingest tranquilizers—presumably because legal guidelines for what may be considered safe blood levels of sedatives have not been established and because of a prevailing lack of awareness among the public that tranquilizers *do* impair concentration. The influence of alcohol, by contrast, is widely publicized.

METHAQUALONE

A more recently popularized sedative drug is methaqualone, a compound marketed by several pharmaceutical companies under such trade names as Parest, Quaalude, Somnafac, and Sopor. Interest in methaqualone has recently been sparked by its use on the street as a "love drug," for it is reputed to be an aphrodisiac and improve sexual performance. Since, pharmacologically, methaqualone is similar to the barbiturates in its effects, it is actually an *an*aphrodisiac. In this instance, it appears that effects of set, setting, and expectations are more potent than the pharmacological effects of the drug.

It should be noted, however, that low doses of any sedative drug can induce relief from anxiety and promote euphoria. The side effects and toxicity of methaqualone are similar to those associated with the barbiturates. Behavior and driving abilities will be impaired and the possibility of the development of tolerance and dependence should be considered. Methaqualone, far from being a "love drug," is merely one of several sedative-hypnotic compounds on the market, all of which may favorably affect the user when administered in the appropriate setting and with the proper mental set or expectations.[2]

GENERAL ANESTHETICS

General anesthesia, a behavioral state on the continuum of depression illustrated in Figure 3.1, is the most severe state of depression intentionally induced pharmacologically. Beyond general anesthesia there are only coma and death. Thus, the induction of general anesthesia with depressant drugs is a serious undertaking and should be performed only by competent persons.

The agents that are used to induce general anesthesia differ widely in physical properties and chemical structure. They range from gases (such as nitrous oxide), to volatile liquids (ether, chloroform, halothane, and so on), to drugs in solutions intended for intravenous administration (thiopental). The gases and volatile liquids are inhaled into the lungs; the other anesthetics are usually injected directly into the bloodstream. All anesthetics are rapidly distributed to the brain, where anesthesia is thought to follow depression of synaptic transmission. The exact mechanisms, however, have not been delineated. It is thought that depression of the arousal center in the brainstem (the ARAS) is involved in the loss of consciousness (see Appendix III).

General anesthetics (like the other sedative-hypnotics) produce a generalized, graded, dose-related depression of all functions of the central nervous system. Thus, the pharmacological effects observed with the general anesthetics are the same as those observed with the barbiturates: an initial period of sedation, relief from anxiety, and disinhibition, followed by onset of sleep. As anesthesia deepens, reflexes are progressively depressed and analgesia is induced. At this point, a patient is said to be anesthetized. Deepening of anesthesia results in loss of reflexes and depression of respiration and of brain excitability: a state of deep anesthesia.

Occasionally, certain anesthetic agents become misused drugs. Nitrous oxide is an example. A gas of low anesthetic potency, it is incapable of inducing deep levels of anesthesia if an adequate oxygen concentration is maintained. Nitrous oxide induces a state of behavioral disinhibition, analgesia, and euphoria. One of the problems occasionally encountered when nitrous oxide is used for recreational purposes is that, unless the compound is administered with at least 20 percent oxygen, hypoxia (decreased oxygen content of the blood) can be induced. But in order to achieve high enough concentrations of nitrous oxide to get a good behavioral effect, concentrations of 50 percent or greater must be inhaled. If such concentrations are mixed with room air, inhaled oxygen concentrations drop to low levels and the hypoxia may result in irreversible brain damage.

Within the last few years other forms of recreational anesthesia with accompanying hypoxia induced by the inhalation of glue, gasoline, and so on have been encountered. The volatile hydrocarbons in these products are capable of inducing a general anesthesia similar to that produced by ether or the other anesthetics. Thus, when these products are administered by people who do not know any better, the dangers of hypoxia or depression of respiration from too deep a level of anesthesia may occasionally result in death. The results of the inhalation of these volatile products, which are found throughout our society, are pharmacologically similar to those of the inhalation or ingestion of any other sedative-hypnotic compound.

MISCELLANEOUS SEDATIVE-HYPNOTIC AGENTS

Table 2.1 in Chapter 2 lists a number of sedative-hypnotic compounds not yet discussed: ethyl alcohol, bromide, paraldehyde, and chloral hydrate. Ethyl alcohol will be discussed in the next chapter, but brief mention should be made of the other agents. All of these compounds, even though they are of diverse chemical structure, have in common that, like barbiturates, they produce a nonspecific, reversible depression of the central nervous system. Their uses and pharmacological effects are similar to the drugs already discussed in this chapter. Some of the agents, however, have a few special properties that deserve mention.

Bromide

Bromide was introduced in 1857 as a depressant of the central nervous system. Being an effective agent for the depression of the CNS, bromide was used in the treatment of epileptic convulsions until the 1900s when the barbiturates were introduced. The mechanism by which bromide depresses the CNS is unknown, but it is thought that it involves a displacement of chloride from the brain. In contrast to the barbiturates, one dose rarely induces acute intoxication. The drug tends to accumulate in the body, however, and chronic bromism is occasionally encountered. It is evidenced by mental disturbances (impaired thought and memory, irritability, emotional disturbances, delirium, delusions, hallucinations, mania, and so on), together with a body rash and other peripheral manifestations. The treatment of chronic bromism is easy: table salt (sodium chloride) is administered in large quantities, and the salt helps the urinary excretion of bromide, which is replaced (in the body) by chloride as a normal consequence of kidney function.

Chloral Hydrate

A number of alcohols are useful as sedative-hypnotic agents. Ethyl alcohol (ethanol) is obviously an important example and is described in the next chapter. However, many other alcohols have been used therapeutically, among them chloral hydrate, ethchlorvynol (Placidyl), paraldehyde, and a few other miscellaneous compounds.

We will not describe their pharmacology here, since it is similar to that of the barbiturates discussed earlier. All these compounds depress the CNS in a manner similar to that of other sedative-hypnotic agents. They are mentioned here merely because they are similar to other general depressant compounds. More detailed descriptions of these alcohols may be found in the textbooks of pharmacology listed in the bibliography.

USE OF SEDATIVE-HYPNOTIC COMPOUNDS IN PREGNANCY

As we pointed out in Chapter 1 (Figure 1.8), drugs are transferred from the mother to the fetus through the placenta. Because the sedative-hypnotic compounds are capable of depressing all systems of the body, their distribution through the placenta implies that they will also depress the fetus. This is a serious problem that at present is not clearly resolved. Very little is known about the effects of depressant drugs on the fetus at the time of delivery, during the developmental years, or later in life. Precisely because of this lack of specific data, caution is necessary. It is known that when sedative-hypnotic agents are administered at the time of delivery, they are found in the newborn baby in significant concentrations, and because the newborn baby has limited metabolizing and excreting systems, it is frequently depressed for a long time after delivery. It would be pharmacologically and medically prudent to avoid the use of sedative-hypnotics either during pregnancy or at the time of delivery, unless the drugs are administered under the close supervision of a physician.

NOTES

1. F. H. Meyers, E. Jawetz, and A. Goldfien, *Review of Medical Pharmacology*, 3d ed. (Los Altos, Calif.: Lange Medical Publications, 1972), p. 219.
2. For a review of methaqualone, see D. R. Wesson and D. E. Smith, "Methaqualone: Just Another Downer," *Journal of Psychedelic Drugs* 5, no. 2 (Winter 1972): 167–69, and H. W. Elliott, ed., "Drugs of Abuse—1973," *Annual Review of Pharmacology* (1974), pp. 517–20.

Chapter 4

Alcohol: The Most Popular Drug

By alcohol we mean ethyl alcohol, a psychoactive drug that is quite as powerful as the more notorious drugs but so accepted in our culture that, for instance, a group gathering to "promote learning and education to end the abuse of drugs" sees no irony in offering cocktails before its fund-raising luncheon.

Ethyl alcohol (alcohol, ethanol) is a drug similar in most respects to the sedative-hypnotic compounds we discussed in the previous chapter. Alcohol is classified pharmacologically as a general depressant and is capable of inducing a general, nonselective, reversible depression of the central nervous system. However, it differs from the compounds discussed in Chapter 3 in that it is used primarily for social or recreational rather than medical purposes. Being one of the most widely used of all drugs, alcohol has created special problems both for the individual user and for society in general. Thus, it deserves separate discussion.

HOW ALCOHOL IS HANDLED BY THE BODY

Alcohol is absorbed, distributed, metabolized, and excreted in certain specific ways.

Absorption

Alcohol is rapidly and completely absorbed from the entire gastrointestinal tract. Already liquid, alcohol does not have to dissolve in the stomach as does a drug in tablet form. Alcohol is a small, fat-soluble molecule that readily penetrates body membranes. If it is vaporized, it can be absorbed readily through the lungs. Because it is so rapidly and completely absorbed when taken orally, the drug is seldom administered intravenously; indeed this might even be dangerous because of its potent depressant action on the nervous system. Fatalities have resulted from inhalation of alcohol through the lungs because the drug is so rapidly absorbed and distributed to the brain, causing a sudden depression of the respiratory control centers in the brainstem.

The absorption rate of alcohol can be modified in various ways. In a person with an empty stomach, approximately 20 percent of a single dose of alcohol is absorbed from the stomach, usually quite rapidly. If the stomach is full, absorption will be delayed. The rate of absorption from the stomach also depends on the volume of fluid in which the alcohol is taken. In general, the more concentrated the alcohol in the stomach, the more rapid the absorption. Thus, diluted alcohol solutions (such as beer) are absorbed more slowly than are more concentrated solutions (such as cocktails, which may contain between 10 and 50 percent alcohol).

Approximately 20 percent of the administered alcohol is absorbed from the stomach. The remaining 80 percent is absorbed, rapidly and completely, from the upper intestine, the limiting factor being the time the stomach takes to empty. Food in the stomach will slow absorption for two reasons: first, by diluting the alcohol and covering some of the stomach membranes through which alcohol would be absorbed, and, second, by prolonging the emptying time. Thus, blood levels of alcohol will increase much faster in an individual who has fasted than in someone who had just eaten a large meal. However, in either case, the alcohol will still be completely absorbed; it is only that in the well-fed individual absorption is delayed.

Distribution

Since alcohol is a small molecule soluble in both water and fat, it is evenly distributed throughout all the fluids of the body and all body tissues, including those of the brain. Since vaporized alcohol may be absorbed through the lungs into the blood, the reverse also holds true: small amounts of alcohol are excreted from the body through the lungs. Indeed, most of us are familiar with the "alcohol breath" that results from exhalation of alcohol. Soluble in both water and fat, alcohol may diffuse into all muscle masses and fat deposits of the body. An obese or a muscular person would be expected to have lower blood levels of alcohol than a lean individual to whom an identical dose of the drug was administered. In other words, the obese or muscular individual would have to ingest more drug than a slender individual would in order to achieve the same level of intoxication. However, because of the peculiar rate of metabolism of alcohol by the body (see the next section), a larger individual would retain the alcohol somewhat longer than would a slender person.

Alcohol is also freely distributed to the fetus and recently a "fetal alcohol syndrome" has been described.[1] Such syndrome consists of rather serious birth defects occurring in 30 to 50 percent of newborns of alcoholic mothers.

Metabolism

Approximately 95 percent of the alcohol that enters the body is metabolized before it is excreted. Metabolism of alcohol usually occurs in the liver, where alcohol is converted to carbon dioxide and water. The small amount of alcohol (5 percent) that is not metabolized is excreted unchanged, primarily in the urine and through the lungs. Metabolically, alcohol has little nutritional value because it provides only calories when metabolized and does not provide the vitamins, minerals, or proteins that are essential for good nutrition.

The rate of metabolism of most drugs in the liver depends on the concentration of the drug in the blood: the higher the concentration of the drug, the faster the rate of metabolism. Alcohol, however, differs in that the rate of metabolism is linear with time and is little affected by variations in the concentration of alcohol in the blood. In the adult, the average rate of metabolism of alcohol is approximately 10 milliliter (one-third ounce) of 100 percent ethanol per hour. Thus, the alcohol contained in about 1 ounce of whiskey (about 33 percent ethanol) is metabolized in one hour. In other words, approximately 4 ounces of whiskey (or 40 ounces of beer) would be metabolized in approximately four to six hours.

This indicates that the rate of metabolism of alcohol is relatively slow, constant, and independent of the amount ingested. If one consumes approximately 1 ounce of whiskey per hour, the blood level of alcohol would remain fairly constant. Thus, if a person ingests more alcohol per hour than is metabolized, blood concentrations will increase. This demonstrates that there is a limit to the amount of alcohol that can be consumed in an hour without a person's becoming drunk as a result of the accumulation of alcohol in the blood.

Factors that may alter the rate of metabolism of alcohol are many and varied but usually not of clinical significance. Alcohol, however, is capable of inducing drug-metabolizing enzymes in the liver, thereby increasing its own rate of metabolism (inducing tolerance) and also the rate of metabolism of other compounds similarly metabolized by the liver (cross tolerance). Although there have been many attempts to develop treatments that might hasten the elimination of alcohol (and therefore reduce the seriousness of acute alcohol intoxication), none has succeeded. There is at present no practical way of increasing the rate of metabolism of alcohol.

Mention should be made here of disulfiram (Antabuse), a drug frequently used to treat chronic alcoholism because it inhibits aldehyde dehydrogenase, an enzyme that carries out a specific step in alcohol metabolism (the metabolism of acetaldehyde to acetate). An earlier step in alcohol metabolism is, however, not blocked. Thus, alcohol is still metabolized to acetaldehyde, which accumulates in the body, making the patient extremely uncomfortable with headache, nausea, vomiting, drowsiness, hangover, and so on. Consequently, alcoholics taking disulfiram find that alcohol makes them feel so dreadful that they are discouraged from drinking. If they refuse to continue taking the drug, treatment often fails.

Excretion

Approximately 95 percent of the alcohol ingested is metabolized to products that eventually are converted to carbon dioxide and water. The remaining 5 percent is excreted unchanged by the kidneys and lungs. Thus, the treatment of acute alcohol intoxication by increasing the rate of urinary excretion is obviously doomed to failure, since so little is removed from the body by this route. It therefore appears that, once alcohol is in the body, the slow, steady rate of metabolism of the drug by the liver is the only way of detoxifying the drug and removing it from the body.

SITES AND MECHANISM OF ACTION

The mechanism of action of alcohol is similar to that of the sedative-hypnotic compounds. Alcohol is a general, nonselective CNS depressant, which means that it depresses all the neurons within the brain. Thus, alcohol is not the stimulant so many think it is. In fact, as we discussed in Chapter 3, alcohol and other sedative-hypnotic drugs can induce a "brain syndrome" characterized by disorientation, mental clouding, impaired memory, decreased judgment, and labile affect. Such a state is often misinterpreted as behavioral stimulation. The behavioral stimulation that results from alcohol is similar to the loss of inhibition and induction of euphoria characteristic of low doses of all sedative-hypnotic drugs. It is postulated that inhibitory synapses are depressed slightly earlier than are excitatory ones. Thus, at low doses, a state of disinhibition or mild euphoria is induced—an effect similar to that of barbiturates. At higher doses, excitatory synapses are depressed, producing a progressive reduction in behavioral activity that leads to sleep, general anesthesia, coma, or death.

It appears that alcohol, like the other sedative-hypnotics, exerts a depressant action on the control centers in the brainstem. Indeed, it is thought by some pharmacologists that alcohol depresses the brainstem at doses that are not sufficient to depress the cerebral cortex. One explanation for drunken behavior is that the higher centers in the cerebral cortex may be released from the inhibitory controls exerted upon them from the brainstem, with a resultant impairment of thought, organization, and motor processes. Low doses of alcohol may produce mild euphoria, but also loss of discrimination, fine movement, memory, concentration, control, and so on. There may be wide fluctuations in mood with frequent emotional outbursts. As the levels of alcohol in the brain are increased, the cerebral cortex is depressed and the state of disinhibition or euphoria is progressively lost. Objective testing has clearly demonstrated that alcohol does *not* increase or improve performance.

PHARMACOLOGICAL EFFECTS ON
THE CENTRAL NERVOUS SYSTEM
AND OTHER ORGANS

The graded depression of synaptic transmission is the prime physiological effect of alcohol. Respiration, although transiently stimulated at low doses of alcohol, is progressively depressed and, at very high blood concentrations, death may result. Like the other sedative-hypnotic compounds, alcohol slows EEG activity toward slow-wave sleep and depresses REM sleep, inhibiting dreaming.

Also like the other sedative-hypnotic compounds, alcohol is anticonvulsant and may suppress epileptic convulsions. However, when alcohol ingestion is stopped, this antiepileptic action may be followed by hyperexcitability that may last for several days. An alcoholic (whether or not he or she is also epileptic) may have seizures when the drug is withdrawn, the seizures peaking approximately 8 to 12 hours after the last dose of the drug. This hyperexcitability indicates that alcohol is to be avoided by epileptics. Finally, it should be stressed that the effects of alcohol, being a sedative-hypnotic compound, are additive with other sedative-hypnotic compounds, resulting in more sedation or greater impairment of driving or other performance than might have been expected.

The effects of alcohol on the circulation and on the heart are minor and will not be elaborated upon. Alcohol does dilate the blood vessels in the skin, producing a warm flush and a decrease in body temperature. Thus, alcohol taken to keep warm when one is exposed to cold weather is pointless and might even be dangerous if it is vital to conserve body heat.

The effects of alcohol on the liver are significant. Alcohol increases the rate of synthesis of fat by the liver. The accumulation of fat is found in the livers both of normal individuals and of alcoholics; whether it is somehow related to the cirrhosis of the liver observed in chronic alcoholism is not known. While it is known that *continued* use of *large* amounts of alcohol may interfere with liver function, *acute* alcoholic intoxication or prolonged use of moderate amounts of alcohol may or may not disrupt liver function.

Alcohol exerts a diuretic effect, increasing the excretion of fluids by affecting the functioning of the kidney, by decreasing action of an antidiuretic hormone, and by the diuretic action simply produced by the large quantities of fluid ordinarily ingested as alcoholic beverages. Alcohol, however, does not appear to harm either the structure or function of the kidney.

Alcohol (like methaqualone and the other sedative-hypnotic drugs) is not an aphrodisiac. In fact, while the behavioral disinhibition induced by low doses of alcohol may cause some loss of restraint, alcohol depresses body function and actually interferes with sexual performance; as Shakespeare wrote, "it provokes the desire, but it takes away the performance" *(Macbeth)*.

PSYCHOLOGICAL EFFECTS

The psychological and behavioral effects of alcohol are similar to those of the sedative-hypnotic agents, and we can add little to the previous discussion, especially since there have been few studies of the effects of alcohol on behavior, in comparison to the numbers of studies conducted with other psychopharmacological agents. In general, the short-term effects of alcohol are primarily restricted to the central nervous system. At low doses, disinhibition occurs and this is followed, with increased dosage, by increases in sedation.

The behavioral reaction to the state of disinhibition is unpredictable and is determined to a large extent by the individual, his or her mental set, and the setting in which the drinking occurs. In one setting a person may be relaxed and euphoric; in another, withdrawn or violent. Mental set and setting become progressively *less* important with increasing doses since sedation dominates and behavioral activity decreases. At low doses that produce a state of disinhibition (perhaps 1 to 3 ounces of whiskey), a person may still function (although in less coordinated fashion) and attempt to drive or otherwise endanger himself and others. As the dose increases (perhaps 4 or more ounces) he or she becomes progressively more incapacitated. There is now convincing data that alcohol intoxication, with its resulting disinhibition, plays a major role in a large percentage of crimes of violence.

Long-term effects may involve many different organs of the body, depending on whether drinking is *moderate* or *heavy.* It appears that long-term ingestion of moderate amounts of alcohol (approximately two martinis a day) produces few physiological, psychological, or behavioral changes in the individual. But long-term ingestion of larger amounts leads to a variety of disorders and discomforts affecting many parts of the body and brain. These disorders may be included within the term *alcoholism.* Alcoholism is characterized by the development of tolerance and dependency (discussed below) and by social connotations.

Alcohol is quite caloric but has little nutritional value. A person may survive for years on a diet of alcohol and not much else but suffer slowly developing vitamin deficiency and nutritional diseases, which may result in gradual physical deterioration. Several articles are listed in the bibliography for readers interested in exploring these aspects of alcoholism in greater detail.

TOLERANCE AND DEPENDENCE

The patterns and mechanisms of the development of tolerance to and physical and psychological dependence upon alcohol are similar to those of all the sedative-hypnotic compounds. The extent of tolerance depends upon the amount, pattern, and extent of alcohol ingestion. Individuals who ingest alcohol only intermittently (on sprees), or more regularly but in moderation, develop little or no tolerance; individuals who regularly ingest large amounts of alcohol develop marked tolerance.

The physical dependence that develops with chronic ingestion of alcohol is such that withdrawal of the drug results in a period of rebound hyperexcitability that may lead to convulsions and even death. Concomitant with this hyperexcitability is a period of tremulousness, with hallucinations, psychomotor agitation, confusion and disorientation, sleep disorders, and a variety of associated discomforts—a syndrome sometimes referred to as *delirium tremens* (DTs, rum fits).

Psychological dependence on alcohol also occurs and, indeed, frequently appears to be socially acceptable. This psychological dependence appears to result from the state of disinhibition, relief from anxiety, and euphoria, so that the use of alcohol becomes a compulsive pleasure. Certainly, this psychological attraction to the drug is a major problem to be considered in the treatment of the alcoholic or, more widely, in attempts to discourage the recreational misuse of alcohol.

SIDE EFFECTS AND TOXICITY

Many of the side effects and toxicities associated with alcohol have already been mentioned, but let us summarize them and expand upon them here. In the acute use of alcohol, behavior is altered as a result of depression of the function of the central nervous system, with the induction of a drug-induced "brain syndrome." This is manifested as a clouded sensorium with disorientation, impaired insight and judgment, and diminished intellectual capabilities. One's affect may be labile, with vulnerability to external stimuli and expressions of anger. In high doses, delusions, hallucinations, and confabulations may be present. Socially, these alterations result in an unpredictable state of disinhibition (drunkenness), alterations in driving performance, and uncoordinated motor behavior.

In chronic alcohol ingestion, a variety of chronic toxicities are observed. In the brain, whereas *acute* intoxication produces a *reversible* brain syndrome secondary to reversible depression of nerve cells, long-term alcohol ingestion may *irreversibly* destroy nerve cells, producing a permanent "brain syndrome" with dementia (Korsakoff's syndrome). The liver may become infiltrated with fat and over a period of time may become cirrhotic (scarred). The digestive system is also affected and one may see pancreatitis (inflammation of the pancreas) and chronic gastritis (inflammation of the stomach) with development of peptic ulcers.

In long-term alcoholism with malnutrition, chronic degeneration may be observed. This consists of a bloated look, flabby muscles, fine tremors, and decreased physical capacity and stamina and increased susceptibility to infections. It should be noted, however, that this state of chronic degeneration is not present in the majority of alcoholics with adequate nutrition. Adequate nutrition, however, does not fully protect the brain, the liver, or the digestive tract.

TREATMENT OF ALCOHOLISM

In a text devoted to the basic principles of drug action, discussion of the treatment of drug problems is a secondary objective. However, since the use and abuse of alcohol is so widespread in our society it seems pertinent to delineate briefly some of the newer concepts relating to alcoholism and its treatment.

Prior to about 1960, alcoholism was seldom considered a medical problem. Individuals were routinely arrested for public drunkenness, denied medical services, and allowed to go through a withdrawal syndrome in the drunk tank of the local jail. It was not until the late 1950s that the American Medical Association (or a minority within that association) recognized the syndrome of alcoholism as an illness. In his book *The Disease Concept of Alcoholism,* published in 1960, E. M. Jellinek presented the hypothesis that alcoholism was a disease.[2] Such labeling served to reduce many of the social stigmata of alcoholism and formed the concept that the deficit in alcoholism lay in an individual who is unable to tolerate the effects of alcohol. To be free of the disease of alcoholism, therefore, the person with this deficiency had totally to abstain from alcohol. This concept also implied that no matter how they became alcoholic, all alcoholics were the same since they all had the same disease. Indeed, this concept underlies the vast majority of current alcoholism treatment programs. As Mann puts it, "alcoholism is a disease which manifests itself chiefly by the uncontrollable drinking of the victim, who is known as an alcoholic."[3]

In contrast to this uniform concept, Pattison postulates that there is no single entity which can be defined as alcoholism and that alcoholism is not a unitary concept but a collection of various signs, symptoms, and behaviors.[4,5] Pattison looks upon alcohol dependence as a health problem (rather than a disease) affecting five areas of life health: (1) drinking health, (2) emotional health, (3) vocational health, (4) social/family health, and (5) physical health. Pattison holds that not all alcohol-dependent persons are impaired in each area of life health nor does impairment in one area necessarily imply impairment in other areas.

For example, a person's drinking health may be severely impaired without much alteration in his or her physical or vocational health, as in the executive with adequate diet and social and family supports. On the other hand, in treatment, drinking health may be solved by total abstinence, yet other life areas such as social/family health and emotional health may not be remedied or may be even worsened. Therefore, different individuals with alcohol problems will exhibit different profiles of impairment in life health problems. As such, different prescriptions for treatment and different levels of expectation for success must be employed for each individual. For example, sobriety may be a reasonable expectation for an individual with minimally impaired life health, while attenuated drinking with modest improvements in health may be all that can be reasonably expected for a more severely impaired alcoholic.

Such individualism may be some distance off, however, since society has just recently looked more favorably upon the alcoholic and in general is just beginning to recognize that each alcoholic should be approached individually in both therapy and reasonable objectives of treatment. The goal of future treatment programs may not *necessarily* be total abstinence from alcohol for every alcoholic, but a reduction in life problems associated with drinking with the objective of reducing these problems to nonproblem levels. The readings in the bibliography are intended to aid the interested reader in pursuing these newer concepts of alcoholism and its treatment.[6]

NOTES

1. J. W. Hanson, K. L. Jones, and D. W. Smith, "Fetal Alcohol Syndrome," *Journal of the American Medical Association* 235 (5 April 1976): 1458–60.

2. E. M. Jellinek, *The Disease Concept of Alcoholism* (New Haven, Conn.: Hillhouse Press, 1960).

3. M. Mann, *New Primer on Alcoholism,* 2d ed. (New York: Holt, Rinehart and Winston, 1968).

4. E. M. Pattison, "The Rehabilitation of the Chronic Alcoholic," in *The Biology of Alcoholism,* vol. 3, B. Kissin and H. Begletier, eds. (New York: Plenum Press, 1974), pp. 587–658.

5. E. M. Pattison, L. Sobel, and L. C. Sobel, *Emerging Concepts of Alcohol Dependence* (New York: Springer-Verlag, 1977).

6. See especially U.S. Department of Health, Education, and Welfare, *Alcohol and Health: Second Special Report to the U.S. Congress* (Washington, D.C.: U.S. Government Printing Office, 1974), pp. 145–59.

Chapter 5

Central Stimulants: From Caffeine to Cocaine

The compounds ordinarily classified as central stimulants are drugs that increase the behavioral activity of an individual. These drugs differ widely in their molecular structures and in their mechanisms of action. Thus, describing a drug as a *stimulant* does not adequately describe the pharmacology of that drug. By contrast, the term *nonselective general depressant* nicely characterizes the pharmacology of a large group of drugs that produce graded, nonselective depression of the central nervous system and the effects illustrated in Figure 3.1 in Chapter 3. No such generalization can be made about central stimulants. The convulsions induced by a stimulant such as strychnine, for example, are very different from the behavioral stimulation and psychomotor agitation induced by a stimulant such as amphetamine.

Table 5.1. Classification of CNS Stimulants

Class	Mechanism of action	Examples
1. Behavioral stimulants	Augmentation of norepinephrine neurotransmitter	Cocaine Amphetamines Methylphenidate (Ritalin) Pemoline (Cylert) Phenmetrazine (Preludin)
2. Clinical antidepressants	a. Blockade of norepinephrine reuptake b. Increased norepinephrine secondary to MAO inhibition	Imipramine (Tofranil) Amitriptyline (Elavil) Tranylcypromine (Parnate)
3. Convulsants	Blockade of inhibitory synapses	Strychnine, picrotoxin, pentylenetetrazol (Metrazol), bicuculline
4. General cellular stimulants	a. Activation of intracellular metabolism b. Stimulation of certain acetylcholine synapses	Caffeine Nicotine (tobacco)

The drugs broadly classified as central stimulants may, however, be subdivided into several groups of agents that, because of similarities in sites and mechanisms of action, may be conveniently discussed together. These drugs are divided into four different classes, each classification being based on a different site or mechanism of action (see Table 5.1).

CLASSIFICATION

The first two groups of central stimulants—behavioral stimulants and clinical antidepressants—have as a common denominator the ability to augment the action of the chemical neurotransmitter norepinephrine. In general, the behavioral stimulants will elevate mood and stimulate behavior in normal individuals, whereas the clinical antidepressants are relatively devoid of pharmacological activity in normal individuals, although they relieve depression and elevate mood in individuals who are psychologically depressed. Examples of behavioral stimulants include cocaine, the many derivatives of amphetamine, methylphenidate (Ritalin), pemoline (Cylert), and phenmetrazine (Preludin). Cocaine and the amphetamines are frequently encountered drugs of abuse. Methylphenidate and pemoline are currently employed in the treatment of hyperkinetic disorders of children. Phenmetrazine (as well as the amphetamines and methylphenidate) has been widely used as an appetite suppressant in the treatment of obesity. Among the clinical antidepressants, two subgroups are noted: those which increase norepinephrine activity through a cocaine-like action of blocking reuptake (imipramine and amitriptyline) and those which increase norepinephrine secondary to inhibiting the enzyme which destroys this neurotransmitter. These actions on the norepinephrine neuron are discussed below and in Appendix II.

The third group of CNS stimulants includes a number of compounds that produce convulsions, usually by blocking inhibitory synapses within the brain and spinal cord. Such convulsants include strychnine, picrotoxin, pentylenetetrazol (Metrazol), and bicuculline.

The fourth group of CNS stimulants consists of two widely used compounds. The first is caffeine, which exerts its CNS stimulant action by acting not at the synapse between neurons but rather by working inside nerve cells to increase their rates of cellular metabolism. The second compound is nicotine, the principal ingredient in tobacco. Nicotine exerts its CNS stimulant action secondary to stimulation of certain acetylcholine synapses both within the brain and in the peripheral nervous system.

BEHAVIORAL STIMULANTS

Cocaine and the amphetamines are generally classified as CNS, psychic, psychomotor, or behavioral stimulants. These compounds elevate mood, induce euphoria, increase alertness, reduce fatigue, and, in high doses, produce irritability, anxiety, and a pattern of psychotic behavior. At low doses, amphetamine evokes an alerting, arousal, or behavioral-activating response not unlike one's normal reaction to an emergency or to stress—a reaction that is not surprising since, structurally, amphetamine closely resembles norepinephrine (NE), a compound for which most of the criteria for a transmitter substance in the brain have been met (see Appendix II). Indeed, the central stimulant actions of both amphetamine and cocaine appear to result from the ability of both compounds to mimic or potentiate the action of NE in the brain.

NE appears to be involved in the behavioral activation associated with the fight/flight/fright response (see Appendix II). Thus, one would predict that increased activity of NE synapses within the brain would result in behavioral activation. Similarly, methylphenidate, pemoline, and phenmetrazine appear to elevate mood, relieve depression, depress appetite, and calm hyperkinetic behavior secondary to their ability to augment the action of NE at the synapse. Clinically, these compounds are widely prescribed as amphetamine substitutes both in the treatment of hyperkinetic behavior in children (methylphenidate and pemoline) and in the treatment of obesity (phenmetrazine).

Thus, because of the importance of NE neurons as sites of action of the behavioral stimulants, it seems pertinent to review the NE neuron as a site of drug action and as a neuron important in emotional behavior.

Norepinephrine Theory of Mania and Depression

In the peripheral nervous system, norepinephrine and its close relative epinephrine (adrenalin) play well-established roles in the body's response to stress and emotion. As part of the fight/flight/fright response, these two transmitters, released from neurons, increase the heart rate and the blood flow to skeletal muscle and reduce the blood flow to stomach, kidney, liver, and other internal organs and in general prepare the body for stress, exertion, or the expression of emotion.

There is very little epinephrine in the brain, although NE is present in large amounts. The specific role of this NE in the brain in the control of emotional disorders is not known, although researchers have advanced an attractive hypothesis that emotional disorders may be correlated with functional excesses or deficits of NE at NE synapses within the brain, that emotional depression may be related to a deficiency of NE within the brain and mania to an excessive amount (Figure 5.1). In other words, NE is proposed as the synaptic transmitter responsible for maintaining behavior on a continuum, with mania and depression at the extremes and normality in the middle. Most of the evidence in favor of this hypothesis is at present indirect and based on the action of pharmacological agents on behavior, on the levels of NE within the brain, and on the relative levels of metabolites of NE found in the urine during periods of mania and depression.

According to this hypothesis, drugs that increase the synaptic action of NE produce degrees of behavioral stimulation related to the concentration of NE at the synapse. Conversely, agents that deplete the brain's store of NE or block NE receptors at the synapse induce depression. In support of this hypothesis, it has been demonstrated that amphetamine, cocaine, and the clinical antidepressants (both the MAO inhibitors and the tricyclic compounds) all increase NE activity.

Behavioral state

Depression ↔ Normal ↔ Behavioral stimulation ↔ Mania

NE levels

Low ⟷ Normal ⟷ Slight excess ⟷ Great excess

Drug	NE levels	Behavior
Amphetamine	Up	Up
Cocaine	Up	Up
MAO inhibitors	Up	Up
Tricyclic compounds	Up	Up
Reserpine	Down	Down
Lithium	Down	Down

Figure 5.1. Outline of the norepinephrine hypothesis of mania and depression.

For example, it has been shown in studies of amphetamine abuse and withdrawal that, when the patients were allowed to administer amphetamine to themselves, they became manic and the metabolic by-products of brain NE were elevated. When the amphetamines were withdrawn abruptly, the metabolites decreased (indicating decreased activity of NE synapses in the brain) and the patients became depressed. As the depression slowly disappeared and the patients returned to normal, there was a gradual increase in the metabolites of NE in the urine, indicating that NE synapses were recovering.

In contrast, reserpine (see Chapter 7) is an antipsychotic drug that depletes NE in the brain, producing behavioral depression that can be severe if enough NE is lost. It has been recently demonstrated that lithium (a compound useful in the treatment of mania) blocks the release of NE from the presynaptic nerve terminal and thus decreases the amount of NE in the synapse and therefore at the receptor. Interestingly, lithium is useful in the management of both mania and depression, rather than just mania. This might seem to be a contradiction of the NE hypothesis of mania and depression, but what appears to happen is that as lithium slowly relieves the periods of mania, the periods of depression (that had previously occurred cyclically with periods of mania) spontaneously disappear. Manic-depressive patients experience wide swings in mood, ranging from deep depression to extreme mania. With the mania relieved, brain levels of NE became more stable and the periods of depression decrease.

Norepinephrine Neurons and Mechanisms of Drug Action

It is now becoming clear that drugs are capable of interfering with a variety of processes associated with synaptic transmission at NE nerve terminals. Amphetamine, cocaine, and the clinical antidepressants appear to exert their behavioral effects secondary to a potentiation of the action of NE at the synapse.

There are at least five ways in which a drug would be capable of potentiating the synaptic action of NE. First, the compound might increase the rate of synthesis of transmitter substance, which is norepinephrine. However, since it is a general pharmacological principle that drugs usually *depress* ongoing processes rather than stimulate reactions, such an action would seem unlikely. Indeed, drug-induced augmentation of the rate of NE synthesis has not been demonstrated.

Second, the compound might potentiate the action of NE by decreasing the rate of its metabolic destruction; that is, it might block the enzymes responsible for the metabolism of the transmitter. This appears to be the mechanism of action of one group of the antidepressant compounds (the monoamine oxidase inhibitors). Monoamine oxidase (MAO) is to be found within the presynaptic nerve terminal and destroys NE. If MAO is blocked, NE concentrations in the nerve terminal increase, making more of the transmitter available for release upon the arrival of an action potential and increasing NE action on the postsynaptic receptor.

Third, a drug might augment the action of NE by inducing the release of NE from presynaptic nerve terminals. This would increase the amount of transmitter available to stimulate the postsynaptic receptors. Amphetamine and methylphenidate are stimulant drugs that induce such release of NE. It has been postulated that this is the primary action responsible for the effect of these drugs on behavior.

Fourth, a drug might prolong the action of NE at its postsynaptic receptor by blocking the active uptake of NE from the synaptic cleft back into the presynaptic nerve terminal. The synaptic action of NE is apparently terminated primarily by the active uptake from the synaptic cleft back into the presynaptic terminal from which the NE was originally released. Such a block of active reuptake appears to be the prime mechanism of action of both cocaine and the tricyclic antidepressants.

Finally, drugs may directly stimulate the postsynaptic NE receptor, mimicking the effect of NE. This is thought to be another action of amphetamine, and is in addition to its ability to induce the release of NE from the presynaptic terminal.

The actions of amphetamine, cocaine, and the clinical antidepressants are summarized in Table 5.2. Despite their varied mechanisms of action, all these drugs appear to relieve depression or induce behavioral stimulation in a manner strongly correlated with their ability to increase the amount of NE at the synapse and bearing out the norepinephrine hypothesis of mania and depression presented in Figure 5.1.

AMPHETAMINE

Amphetamine is, structurally, closely related to norepinephrine (see Figure 5.2) and it appears to mimic and potentiate the synaptic action of NE both in the central nervous system and in the rest of the

Table 5.2. Potentiation of Transmission at Norepinephrine Synapses by Various Drugs

Drug	Action
Amphetamine	Increase release of NE Direct stimulation of postsynaptic NE receptors
Methylphenidate	Increase release of NE Direct stimulation of postsynaptic NE receptors
Cocaine	Block of reabsorption of NE by presynaptic nerve terminal
Tricyclic antidepressants	Block of reabsorption of NE by presynaptic nerve terminal
MAO-inhibiting antidepressants	Inhibition of enzyme MAO

body. Amphetamine was first synthesized in the early 1900s, but did not enter medical use until the early 1930s, when it was found that the drug increased blood pressure, stimulated the central nervous system, caused bronchodilatation (useful in treating asthma), and was useful in treating an epileptic seizure disorder called narcolepsy (a disorder in which the patient repeatedly lapses into sleep). Since then, amphetamines have been used for a wide variety of clinical conditions and more recently in a variety of recreational situations.[1]

The most common amphetamine derivatives currently available are amphetamine (Benzedrine), dextroamphetamine (Dexedrine), and methamphetamine (Methedrine or Desoxyn). Other chemicals are available that are structurally related to amphetamine and that share

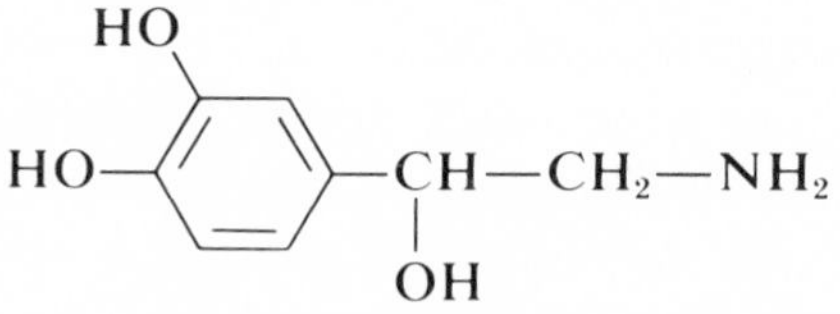

Norepinephrine

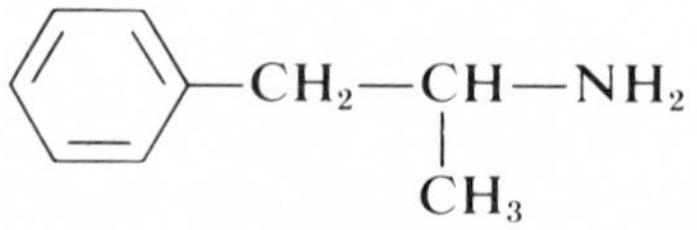

Amphetamine

Figure 5.2. Structural formulas of norepinephrine and amphetamine.

amphetamine's profile of action—for example, phenmetrazine (Preludin), a compound promoted as an appetite suppressant. Despite variances in potency (compensated for by an adjustment in dose), the effects of the amphetamine derivatives are similar to those of amphetamine itself and therefore amphetamine will be discussed at length and the other drugs compared with it.

Therapeutic Uses and Status

The primary *medical* uses of amphetamine are restricted today. Amphetamine was first found useful and specific in the treatment of narcolepsy and is also used to treat a form of epilepsy called petit mal epilepsy.

Amphetamine appears to be useful in the treatment of certain hyperkinetic disorders in children. The hyperkinetic state was originally defined as *minimal brain damage* (MBD). However, the majority of children so diagnosed had no recognizable brain damage. Thus, the newer terms *minimal brain dysfunction* and *hyperkinetic syndrome* have been coined.

The use of amphetamine, and more recently the amphetamine derivatives methylphenidate (Ritalin) and pemoline (Cylert), in the treatment of hyperkinesis is recognized. These drugs improve both behavior and learning ability in 50 to 75 percent of children correctly diagnosed as exhibiting behavioral hyperkinesis. However, indiscriminate use of these behavioral stimulants for "problem children" and sole dependence on drug therapy for minimal brain dysfunction should be discouraged. Many clinicians feel that large numbers of children diagnosed as having minimal brain dysfunction are incorrectly diagnosed and should not be treated with stimulants. In addition, if one carefully examines the family situation of children diagnosed as hyperkinetic, one finds frequently occurring episodes of depression in one or more parents. It has been hypothesized that the hyperkinetic behavior exhibited by the child is a natural defense mechanism against his own state of depression. Such behavior may therefore be considered as a symptom of a deeper problem and not as a disease. Before these compounds are prescribed, therefore, there should be a careful search for signs of depression both in the child and in the parents. Even if the drug corrects the behavioral and learning problems, the home situation should still be explored. Once the causes of depression both in the child and in the family are recognized and alleviated, perhaps at that time drug therapy can be discontinued.

Why amphetamine, methylphenidate, and pemoline (all behavior stimulants) work to calm hyperactive children is not clear. However, if hyperkinesis is a defense against emotional depression, use of an antidepressant drug would serve to alleviate the behavioral symptoms. On the other hand, by increasing attention and learning abilities, a child's anxieties may be relieved and the anxious state is replaced by a state characterized as more pleasant and productive. Indeed, adults in certain anxiety states (such as studying for final examinations) often find that they become more calm and can work more efficiently after taking amphetamine or other stimulants.

To date the above uses of amphetamine are the only ones recognized as clinically significant. The amphetamines, however, have a strong suppressant action on appetite and have been sold extensively as "diet pills." Tolerance to the appetite-suppressant action of amphetamines appears within about two weeks, however, so the dose must be increased. Once tolerance develops, and unless the dose is increased (usually to the point at which the patient becomes agitated), the patient usually resumes his or her previous eating habits and gains back all the weight lost earlier. As a result, amphetamines are no longer recognized as effective drugs for the long-term control of obesity. The federal government is currently considering limiting the availability of amphetamines for use in the treatment of obesity.

Outside medicine, amphetamines are used for many and varied reasons but usually because they are euphoriant or because they improve performance. Characteristically, amphetamines produce a state of euphoria, an action that may largely explain the wide misuse of the drug. As one pharmacology text states, "Since the amphetamines are only transiently effective in treating obesity . . . it must be concluded that most of the five billion doses of diet pills made in the U.S.A. each year are actually used as euphoriants."[2]

It has been well documented that psychomotor, intellectual, or athletic performance may be improved to a slight but statistically significant degree by amphetamines. It is most likely that such improvements are a result of the increased availability of norepinephrine, which will augment alertness and the fight/flight/fright reactions. The amphetamines also have the ability to produce prolonged periods of wakefulness, allaying sleep and inducing insomnia, an action that has been postulated to result from an increase in norepinephrine in the reticular formation, especially in the ARAS, that stimulates the centers responsible for maintaining wakefulness.

Amphetamine and many amphetamine derivatives are widely available legally and illegally in a variety of forms, mixtures, and concoctions. In the legal market, there is probably no area of medicine in which one group of drugs has been so misused. The amphetamines are commercially found mixed with barbiturates, other sedatives, atropine, caffeine, vitamins, thyroid, and numerous other drugs, usually in irrational combinations. For example, in the Le Dain report in Canada, it was stated that one amphetamine combination was described by its manufacturer as follows: "This is a multi-coated tablet of pentobarbital on the outside to induce sleep rapidly, phenobarbital under a delayed dissolving coating to extend the sleep, and under another coating, an amphetamine to awaken a patient in the morning."[3]

As another example of misleading information about amphetamine action, during the period of explosive increases in amphetamine use and abuse in the 1950s and 1960s, it was felt by many that children should not be placed on long-term amphetamine therapy for hyperkinetic disorders, even though many physicians prescribed it. Therefore, two "nonamphetamine" stimulants, methylphenidate (Ritalin) and pemoline (Cylert), were introduced for the treatment of these children. As Figure 5.3 shows, methylphenidate and pemoline are structurally so similar to amphetamine that they probably work on the same receptors in the brain as does amphetamine. Thus, de-

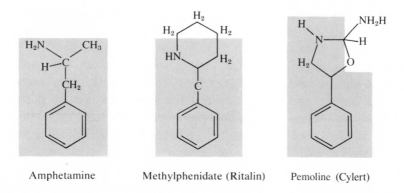

Amphetamine   Methylphenidate (Ritalin)   Pemoline (Cylert)

Figure 5.3. Structural formulas of amphetamine, methylphenidate, and pemoline. This shows the close structural similarities among these drugs. Shading indicates the common portions of the molecules.

spite the fact that methylphenidate and pemoline are *chemically* not amphetamine (which is a chemical term), pharmacologically their effect is virtually identical.

Pharmacological Effects

The physiological responses to amphetamine vary markedly with the dose of the drug. In general, however, we may categorize these into those that are observed at low to moderate doses (5 to 50 mg of amphetamine, usually administered orally) and those that are observed at high doses (doses above approximately 100 mg, often administered intravenously). These dosage ranges are not the same for all amphetamines. For example, dextroamphetamine is more potent than amphetamine. Low to moderate doses of dextroamphetamine would range from 2.5 to 20 mg, while high doses are considered to be those of 50 mg or more. Methamphetamine ("speed") is even more potent, and doses have to be lowered even further.

At *normal, oral* doses, all of the amphetamines induce a significant increase in blood pressure, with a reflex slowing of heart rate, a relaxation of bronchial muscle, and a variety of other responses that are predictable from drugs that mobilize norepinephrine and thus induce the fight/flight/fright response (that is, increased blood sugar, increased blood flow to musculature, decreased blood flow to internal organs, dilation of pupils, increased rate of respiration, and so on). In the central nervous system, the amphetamines are potent stimulants, producing both EEG and behavioral signs of increased alertness and excitement. Athletic performance is enhanced.[4]

At moderate doses (5 to 50 mg), effects of amphetamine in the brain include stimulation of respiration, production of a slight tremor, restlessness, increased motor activity, insomnia, and agitation. In addition, amphetamine prevents fatigue, suppresses appetite, and promotes wakefulness. The wakefulness is of interest since even with amphetamines the biological need for sleep may not be postponed indefinitely. When the administration of amphetamines is stopped, there is a rebound increase in sleep time. Indeed, such drug-induced sleep deficits, with subsequent rebound, are significant and complete recovery of normal sleeping patterns may take many weeks.

During chronic use of amphetamine in high doses (100 mg or more), a different pattern of physiological effects is observed, partly because such high doses are usually administered intravenously. Daily doses in the range of 100 mg to several grams have been reported.

During prolonged, high-dose "sprees," an individual experiences a paranoid mania that is induced both by the excessive levels of NE (Figure 5.1) and by the chronic lack of sleep and food. In addition, the intravenous injection of the drug provides a sudden "flash" or "rush," described by users as being extremely pleasurable and very similar to an intensive whole-body sexual orgasm. These pleasurable effects, however, are offset by the manic paranoia that is induced. Withdrawal of the drug and subsequent termination of the "spree" is followed by fatigue. Deep sleep occurs and may last for several days. Upon awakening, the user is lethargic, emotionally depressed, and intensely hungry. Food and counseling may be helpful in this withdrawal period or the user may try more injections of amphetamine, thus initiating another spree.

Psychological Effects

The psychological effects of the amphetamines differ widely depending upon the dose administered. At low to moderate doses, an individual typically experiences increased alertness, wakefulness, elevation of mood, mild euphoria, increased athletic performance, decreased fatigue, possible freedom from boredom, less mental clouding, clearer thinking, improvements in concentration, increased energy and, in general, increased levels of behavioral activity. All of this is in agreement with the role of norepinephrine in behavioral alerting or arousal responses. Some of the effects of these low doses may be bothersome, for they include increased irritability, restlessness and insomnia, blurred vision, increased blood pressure, cardiac palpitations, and anxiety. Occasionally, aggression, hallucinations, and psychosis may occur, although these are usually the effects of higher doses.

High-dose intravenous use induces a pattern of psychosis that may be indistinguishable from schizophrenia. One observes confused and disorganized behavior, compulsive repetition of meaningless acts, irritability, fear, suspicion of everything and everyone, hallucinations, and delusions. The user may become aggressive and extremely antisocial. Also, whole-body orgasm may be induced, a pleasure that may be the major attraction of the drug. In addition, since these high doses are usually administered by injection, a factor to be considered is the attraction of certain individuals to the hypodermic needle. Such individuals derive pleasure from the intravenous injection of various substances, and may even inject ice water when psychoactive drugs are not available. The basis for this attraction is not known, but the transient "rush" or "flash" set up by spasms in the heart and the blood vessels of the brain and other parts of the body is possibly involved.

Side Effects and Toxicity

The side effects induced by low doses of amphetamine are usually extensions of the drug's behavioral actions: restlessness and tremor, anxiety, insomnia, dizziness, irritability, and tenseness. These side effects are usually tolerable and decrease within a few days as tolerance develops. Amphetamines also increase blood pressure and may cause heart palpitations. Sweating, a dry mouth, and nausea and vomiting may also occur. Fatalities are rare.

The side effects of prolonged use of high doses are more serious and usually seen only when amphetamines are abused because there is no medical justification for the prolonged use of high doses of amphetamines. Psychosis and abnormal mental conditions similar to those observed in schizophrenia are common, together with considerable weight loss, skin sores, infections resulting from neglected health care, and a variety of other consequences of the drug itself or of poor eating habits, lack of sleep, and the use of unsterile equipment for intravenous injections.

However, fatalities directly attributable to the use of amphetamine are rare. Individuals who have no tolerance have survived doses of 400 to 500 mg. Even larger doses are tolerated by chronic users. What then is the evidence for the slogan "speed kills"? It appears that this expression does not refer literally to a direct effect of single doses of amphetamine, but to the deteriorating mental and physical condition and the destructive and aggressive behavior induced by prolonged high-dose amphetamine sprees. Such sprees are detrimental to both the mental and the physical health of the individual and often to those with whom he interacts. Only rarely does even high-dose, intravenous use of amphetamine result in lethal rupture of blood vessels as a result of drug-induced increases in arterial pressure. Thus, rather than implying that amphetamines are lethal compounds, the slogan appears to refer to the drug-induced "death" of the mind, spirit, or personality of the user.

Dependence

Dependence on the sedative-hypnotic compounds has been described as consisting of two components: psychological and physiological. Psychological dependence is described as a compulsion to use a drug repeatedly for its enjoyable effects. The euphoric or pleasurable state that follows even moderate doses of amphetamine and the drug-induced "rush" and orgasm that may be induced by intravenous use of the drug can lead to a compulsion to misuse the drug.

Physiological dependence to the sedative-hypnotic compounds has been described as as a period of rebound hyperexcitability following withdrawal of the drug. Withdrawal of amphetamine produces, not the hyperexcitability associated with the sedative-hypnotic drugs, but fatigue, profound and prolonged sleep, EEG changes characteristic of sleep, severe emotional depression, and increased appetite. This certainly is not unexpected; one would predict that, if the body and the brain were continually stimulated by amphetamine, such stimulation would be followed by depression upon removal of the drug.

Tolerance

Tolerance to the many effects of amphetamine develops at different rates and to different degrees, and tolerance to some effects may never develop. Tolerance of the appetite-suppressing effect of amphetamine almost invariably develops, and this is the principal reason that these compounds usually fail to be effective in the long-term treatment of obesity. The mood-elevating action of amphetamine is subject to tolerance but not to quite the same extent as the appetite-suppressant effect. Tolerance to the peripheral effects of amphetamines also develops, so that a habitual user of amphetamine is able to increase the dose considerably in order to attain a desired effect as his or her tolerance to the central effects builds. Yet there are some effects of amphetamine to which tolerance does not develop at all. For instance, in the treatment of narcolepsy and hyperactivity, once an adequate controlling dose is achieved, there may be little need to increase the dose of amphetamine for many years.

COCAINE

Cocaine is a behavioral stimulant that inhibits the active reuptake of norepinephrine into presynaptic nerve terminals (Table 5.2) in the brain and the peripheral nervous system. It is thought that this blockage increases the amount of NE in the synaptic cleft, thereby increasing the synaptic action of NE—the mechanism by which cocaine stimulates the central nervous system.

Cocaine is also an extremely potent local anesthetic. Nerve endings are anesthetized whenever they come into contact with the drug. Thus, when cocaine is sniffed, the compound anesthetizes the nerve endings in the nose.

Cocaine increases the heart rate and constricts blood vessels (increasing blood pressure). Cocaine also relaxes the muscles of the bronchial airways of the lung, and because the blood vessels of the nose are constricted, it makes for easier breathing. But when the drug wears off, the bronchial muscles contract and the blood vessels relax, so that regular users of cocaine suffer from nasal stuffiness and tender, bleeding nasal membranes. As a result, a cocaine user will often obtain relief by sniffing more drug, delaying but intensifying the symptoms. Also, owing to the swollen nasal membranes and the accompanying stuffiness, the user may tend to blow or rub his or her nose frequently, thus setting up further irritation and inflammation.

In the central nervous system, cocaine is a powerful stimulant. The cortex is affected first and then the brainstem. Thus, mental awareness and abilities are increased, but muscular strength is not, and the sense of fatigue is decreased. Behaviorally, cocaine increases motor activity, which becomes less and less coordinated as the dose is increased and the brainstem centers that coordinate movement are affected by the drug.

In general, the syndrome of behavioral and toxic effects (including paranoia) produced by cocaine is similar to that produced by amphetamine—a similarity that would be expected, considering the similar sites of action of amphetamine and cocaine on NE nerve terminals, resulting in potentiation of norepinephrine. As with amphetamine, respiration and heart rate are stimulated and vomiting may be induced. Withdrawal from cocaine is followed by profound physical and emotional depression similar to that occasioned by withdrawal from amphetamine.

One significant difference, however, between cocaine and amphetamine is in the duration of action. Whereas the effects of amphetamine may last for several hours, cocaine may be active in the body for only a few minutes because it is metabolized by the liver extremely rapidly. A dose of cocaine may be metabolized in 5 to 15 minutes. Thus, except for their different time courses of action and the fact that cocaine is also a powerful local anesthetic, the pharmacology of cocaine closely resembles that of amphetamine.

Cocaine taken orally is poorly absorbed (although a little antacid may aid gastrointestinal absorption) and intravenous use is extremely dangerous and possibly lethal because the drug is so potent.

There are at present few medical uses for cocaine. The close similarity of cocaine to amphetamine and the ability of both compounds to potentiate norepinephrine appear to be responsible for the interest in the drug. Both cocaine and amphetamine are potent central stimulants, increasing performance and inducing euphoria, a feeling of well-being, power, and boundless energy. Cocaine, like amphetamine, causes tolerance, psychological dependency, and physiological dependence.

The social misuse of cocaine is not new. In 1884, Sigmund Freud advocated use of cocaine for relief from depression and chronic fatigue, describing it as a "magical drug." He wrote the "Song of Praise" to cocaine, which was published in 1884. In relieving his own depression, Freud described small doses of cocaine as inducing "exhilaration and lasting euphoria, which in no way differs from the normal euphoria of the healthy person."[5] Freud, however, did not immediately perceive the liability of cocaine to produce tolerance, dependency, a state of psychosis, and withdrawal depression.

As amphetamine became available in the 1930s, the use of cocaine diminished, probably because amphetamine cost less and lasted longer. Thus, cocaine was little used until the late 1960s, when tight federal restrictions on amphetamine distribution raised the cost of amphetamine to the point where cocaine was once again attractive.[6] Because their actions at the NE synapse are similar, cocaine and amphetamine can be used almost interchangeably as euphoriants, so their use and popularity in the future will most likely be determined by availability and price. Brecher presents an interesting discussion of the role of the federal government and its narcotic agents in the popularity, availability, and price of drugs.[7]

CLINICAL ANTIDEPRESSANTS

Earlier in this chapter, we mentioned that the clinical antidepressants (the MAO inhibitors and the tricyclic compounds) were compounds that are capable of elevating mood in depressed patients. The MAO inhibitors inhibit the enzyme monoamine oxidase, and thereby increase levels of norepinephrine within NE neurons. The tricyclic compounds exert a cocainelike effect on the presynaptic nerve terminal, blocking active reuptake of NE into the terminal, thus potentiating NE action at the synapse. It therefore appears that both the MAO inhibitors and the tricyclic antidepressants owe their antidepressant action to potentiation of the synaptic action of NE. Their prime uses are in the medical treatment of depression.

These drugs are potent and should be used only under close medical supervision. This applies particularly to the MAO inhibitors, of which tranylcypromine (Parnate) is an example. It was found a few years ago that hypertensive crises and deaths occurred in a number of patients on tranylcypromine. These patients showed a common liking for certain aged cheeses (especially cheddar, Camembert, and Stilton) that were rich in substances that could cause the release of NE. Apparently, since the tranylcypromine had inactivated the enzyme that destroys NE, there was no way for the body to modulate the action of NE and drastic increases in blood pressure and several fatalities resulted. Subsequently, other foods were implicated in this syndrome, among them aged wine, pickled herring, and sardines.

Complete pharmacologic descriptions of the MAO inhibitors and the tricyclic antidepressants may be found in the textbooks of pharmacology listed in the bibliography. We mention these compounds to reinforce the concept that various drugs are capable of stimulating the CNS and increasing NE activity. In addition, the actions of these drugs add further evidence to support the NE theory of mania and depression. The reason that these compounds, unlike amphetamine and cocaine, have not become drugs of abuse appears to be because neither the MAO inhibitors nor the tricyclic compounds influence behavior in *normal* individuals; only the depressed patient is affected by these drugs.

EPHEDRINE, METARAMINOL, PHENYLEPHRINE, METHOXAMINE, AND OTHERS

There are many drugs structurally related either to amphetamine or to norepinephrine that are capable of altering the synaptic action of NE both in the brain and in the periphery. Some of these agents release NE from presynaptic terminals; others directly stimulate postsynaptic NE receptors. Despite this difference in exact site of action, however, these compounds have the inherent ability to induce a pattern of physiological and behavioral responses similar to those induced by amphetamine, although the central effects of some of these agents are mild and high doses might be required. Their number is bewildering, but perhaps their names might be mentioned because many are likely to be familiar to the reader.

Representative products include ephedrine, mephentermine (Wyamine), metaraminol (Aramine), phenylephrine (Neo-Synephrine), methoxamine (Vasoxyl), methoxyphenamine (Orthoxine), nylidrin (Arlidin), propylhexedrine (Benzedrex), phenmetrazine (Preludin), naphazoline (Privine), and oxymetazoline (Afrin). These compounds differ from one another primarily in the intensity of their effects on the body (heart rate, breathing, and the like) and in the degree to which they stimulate behavior. In general, the responses to these drugs are similar to those observed for amphetamine, except most have very poor CNS effects. Many of these drugs are used as nasal decongestants and they produce rebound increases in nasal stuffiness when the drug action wears off, a response similar to the stuffy nose induced by cocaine.

CONVULSANTS

There are many different drugs that exert a generalized stimulant action on the central nervous system and that are capable of inducing convulsions when administered in sufficient quantity. Notable examples are strychnine, picrotoxin, pentylenetetrazol, and bicuculline. These compounds differ from the drugs discussed earlier in this chapter in that they do *not* exert their effects through the NE synapses and therefore do not produce the continuum of behavioral states illustrated in Figure 5.1. These compounds stimulate principally the spinal cord and brainstem and have, in general, less effect on the cerebral cortex. Although seldom clinically useful, the convulsants can stimulate respiration, temporarily counteract the action of depressant drugs, induce hyperactive spinal-cord reflexes, and, in general, increase the excitability of the nervous system without markedly augmenting the higher functions of the cerebral cortex (such as creativity or thinking ability).

The general rule that most pharmacological agents exert their effects secondary to a blockade of on-going activity applies to the convulsants. The behavioral stimulation, hyperactivity, and convulsions that they induce occur as a result of their blocking inhibitory synapses in the spinal cord and the brainstem, which has the overall effect of markedly increasing the excitability of the central nervous system. As might be expected, these convulsant agents are not considered drugs of any useful therapeutic value. One would also question their recreational value, since they merely increase excitability without concomitant production of euphoria or augmentation of cortical function. Despite this, these drugs are occasionally encountered in illicit drug preparations, presumably as unwanted replacements for cocaine or amphetamine.

Administration, orally or (especially) intravenously, is extremely dangerous. They may induce powerful convulsions, which can disrupt the brainstem and, consequently, paralyze respiration, leading ultimately to cardiac arrest and death. In addition, since the action of stimulant drugs is followed by behavioral depression, profound CNS depression is observed during recovery from these agents. The drugs are so gross in their action on the nervous system that, once they have been administered, treatment of overdose is nonspecific and not very effective because there are no specific antidotes. About all one is able to do is to prevent convulsions and support respiration. Convulsions can be prevented with a sedative-hypnotic drug, but when the convulsant is metabolized and the patient becomes depressed, the sedative-hypnotic deepens the depression, further endangering the patient.

CAFFEINE

Caffeine is one of the most widely used stimulants in the world, being found in significant concentrations in coffee, tea, cola drinks, chocolate candy, and cocoa. The average cup of coffee contains between 100 and 150 mg of caffeine, and a 12-ounce bottle of a cola drink contains between 35 and 55 mg. Even in chocolate bars, the caffeine content may be as high as 25 mg per ounce. It has been estimated that the annual consumption of caffeine in the United States in the form of coffee alone is about 15 million pounds.

The main pharmacological actions of caffeine are exerted on the CNS, the heart, the kidneys, the lungs, and the arteries supplying blood to the heart and brain. Most of these actions appear to be the result of caffeine-induced augmentation of the rates of cellular metabolism. Current thought holds that this action is exerted through a chemical substance called cyclic adenosine monophosphate (cyclic AMP). Caffeine inhibits an enzyme that ordinarily breaks down cyclic AMP to its inactive end-product. The resultant increase in cyclic AMP leads to increased glucose production within cells and thus makes available more energy to allow higher rates of cellular activity.

Absorption, Distribution, Metabolism, and Excretion

Caffeine, existing in the stomach primarily in a water-soluble form, is only slowly and incompletely absorbed into the bloodstream. Thus, absorption is delayed and occurs largely through the intestine.

As a result, caffeine is absorbed slowly (only approximately 25 percent in one hour), but completely.

Goldstein, Aronow, and Kalman have demonstrated that caffeine is freely and equally distributed throughout the total body water and, indeed, is distributed across the placenta into the fetus.[8] (This latter point is significant and the implications will be discussed below.) Thus, caffeine is found in almost equal concentrations in all parts of the body, including the brain. Most of the caffeine is metabolized by the liver before it is excreted by the kidneys. Only approximately 10 percent of the drug is excreted unchanged (that is, without being metabolized).

Pharmacological Effects

In the brain, caffeine is a powerful stimulant of nerve tissue. The cortex, being most sensitive, is affected first, followed next by the brainstem. The spinal cord becomes stimulated last and only after extremely high doses of the drug. Since the cerebral cortex is affected at doses lower than those necessary to excite the brainstem, the earliest behavioral effects of caffeine are increases in mental alertness, a more rapid and clearer flow of thought, wakefulness, and restlessness. This increased mental awareness may result in sustained intellectual effort for prolonged periods without the disruption of coordinated intellectual or motor activity that usually follows alteration of the function of the medulla (as occurs with amphetamine, cocaine, or the convulsants). These effects on the cerebral cortex may be observed after oral doses of as little as 100 or 200 mg of caffeine, the amount of the drug that is contained in one to two cups of coffee.

Only after massive doses (probably 2 to 5 grams) is the spinal cord stimulated by caffeine. Increased excitability of spinal reflexes might be observed and, at even higher doses, convulsions and death may ensue. The convulsive dose, however, is so high (over 10 grams, the equivalent of 100 cups of coffee) that death from caffeine is highly unlikely.

Caffeine has a slight stimulant action on the heart, resulting in increased cardiac contractility, with an increase in the total amount of blood pumped by the heart per minute (increased cardiac output). Caffeine also affects the arteries supplying blood to the heart (the *coronary* arteries), causing their dilation. This increases the flow of oxygenated blood to the heart muscle and increases the work capability of the heart. It should be noted, however, that caffeine *decreases* blood flow to the brain by constricting the cerebral blood vessels.

Such action affords striking relief from headaches associated with increased blood pressure (hypertensive headaches) and provides some relief of certain types of migraine headaches, conditions for which caffeine is used clinically.

Another action of caffeine is to relax the musculature of the bronchi of the lungs, although a closely related compound, theophylline is more potent in this regard. Caffeine also exerts a diuretic effect on the kidney, although therapeutic efficacy as a useful diuretic might be questioned.

Psychological Effects

In normal doses (100 to 500 mg), caffeine potently stimulates the cerebral cortex, promoting wakefulness and improving psychomotor performance. The stimulation, however, is not nearly as great as that induced by amphetamine. It must be remembered that once any stimulant agent is metabolized, there follows a period of behavioral and mental depression. This may be expressed frequently in automobile accidents that may occur as a result of people driving for prolonged periods under caffeine stimulation. If people stop drinking coffee, they may become drowsy and fall asleep while driving. Such depression should be considered when any of the stimulant drugs (such as amphetamine, cocaine, or caffeine) are ingested to maintain wakefulness or performance for prolonged periods.

Side Effects

The side effects associated with the use of caffeine are extensions of its primary effect. One frequently observes periods of wakefulness and insomnia, psychomotor agitation, increases in heart rate with occasional arrhythmias, and either increases or decreases in blood pressure (usually not of great significance). With higher doses of the drug, mild delirium may be induced.

Dependence and Tolerance

With the usually administered doses of caffeine, little tolerance of the central stimulant actions develops. Some slight tolerance, however, may develop after prolonged ingestion of larger doses. It appears that caffeine does not induce physiological dependence (that is, dependence characterized by withdrawal syndromes). However, as many millions of individuals can attest, some degree of psychological dependence on beverages containing caffeine may develop. Many of us "need" our coffee to get going in the morning, but there is no evidence to indicate that this psychological dependence is harmful.

Teratogenesis and Mutagenesis

Certain drugs endanger the fetus when they are ingested during pregnancy. Such toxicities are usually manifested as either mutagenesis (changes in the genetic code) or teratogenesis (abnormal development). Goldstein, Aronow, and Kalman point out that caffeine may induce chromosomal breakage in a variety of nonmammalian species.[9] Indeed, caffeine is used as a laboratory standard for studies of chromosomal breakage. The doses required to induce such breakage, however, are significantly higher than those usually consumed by humans.

It does not appear at this time that ingestion of tea or coffee increases mutation rate in humans, and most researchers have concluded, therefore, that caffeine does not constitute a *significant* toxic hazard to the fetus. One note of caution, however, was expressed by Goldstein, *et al.:* "Caffeine should be regarded as possibly hazardous to the fetus during the first three months of pregnancy."[10] Such caution is warranted whenever *any* drug is ingested, especially a widely used drug that is freely distributed throughout the body and that easily crosses the placenta.

NICOTINE

Next to caffeine, nicotine, an active ingredient in tobacco, is the most widely used psychoactive agent in our society. Despite the fact that nicotine currently has little therapeutic application in medicine, its extreme potency and widespread use affords a considerable amount of importance to this compound, especially as recent evidence indicates a wide range of toxicity in both nicotine and other ingredients of tobacco. Since the present discussion concerns the pharmacological properties of psychoactive drugs, the reader is referred to Brecher for a history of tobacco.[11]

Absorption, Distribution, Metabolism, and Excretion

Nicotine is readily and completely absorbed from the stomach after oral administration and from the lungs upon inhalation. Most cigarettes contain between 1 and 10 mg of nicotine, depending upon the brand. Conservative estimates would indicate that approximately 10 percent (between 0.1 and 0.3 mg) of this nicotine will actually be inhaled and absorbed into the bloodstream. Indeed, the physiological effects of smoking a single cigarette can be closely duplicated by the intravenous injection of these amounts of nicotine. This is well below the lethal dose of the drug, which is considered to be approximately 60 mg.

Like most psychoactive drugs, nicotine is quickly and ubiquitously distributed, rapidly penetrating the brain, all body organs, the fetus, and, in general, all body fluids.

Approximately 80 to 90 percent of the nicotine that is administered to an individual either orally or by smoking must be metabolized by the liver before it can be excreted by the kidneys. Nicotine is also excreted in the milk of lactating women who smoke. Indeed, the breast-fed infant may have a blood level of nicotine which may be as high as or even higher than that of the mother. It is not clear at this time whether such infants suffer adverse consequences nursing from a mother who smokes. The passage of nicotine through breast milk is, however, cause for concern.

Pharmacological Effects

Nicotine is an extremely potent compound exerting powerful effects on the brain, the spinal cord, the peripheral nervous system, the heart, and various other body structures. Pharmacologically, nicotine appears to exert this action secondary to a direct stimulation of certain receptors sensitive to the transmitter acetylcholine. This stimulation of acetylcholine receptors is manifested as CNS stimulation, increased blood pressure, increased heart rate, release of epinephrine (adrenalin) from the adrenal glands (inducing symptoms characteristic of the fight/flight/fright response), and increased tone and activity of the gastrointestinal tract.

Nicotine appears to stimulate the central nervous system at all levels, including the cerebral cortex, producing increased levels of behavioral activity. The drug is capable of inducing tremors and, in large doses, convulsions. As with all stimulant drugs, stimulation of the brain is followed by a period of depression. Nicotine is also capable of stimulating the vomiting and the respiratory centers in the brainstem. It stimulates the hypothalamus to release a hormone called ADH (antidiuretic hormone), which causes an individual to retain fluid because the excretion of urine is reduced. The effect of nicotine on nerve fibers coming from the muscles leads to a marked reduction in muscle tone and may be involved (at least partially) in the relaxation that can accompany smoking.

In addition to their effects on the central nervous system, normal doses of nicotine are capable of increasing heart rate and blood pressure and stimulating the heart muscle. Nicotine also increases blood flow to the heart and to skeletal muscle. Because nicotine also increases the tone and activity of the bowel, it may occasionally induce diarrhea.

Psychological Effects

The primary psychological effects of nicotine consist of mild to moderate stimulation of the central nervous system. To date, the effects of nicotine on behavioral performance have not been elucidated, although there is evidence in animals that nicotine will increase motor activity.

In humans, nicotine appears to induce some degree of psychological dependence. Such dependence is evidenced by the strong compulsion of many cigarette smokers to continue smoking. The precise basis for this compulsion is not known, but it is quite clear that it is related to the nicotine content of the tobacco, since nicotine-free tobacco can seldom be substituted for ordinary cigarettes.

Whether physiological dependence on nicotine can develop is not clear, although individuals who have attempted to stop smoking have experienced withdrawal effects apparently uncomfortable enough to make them revert to their previous smoking habits. Exactly how much of this compulsion to return to smoking is due to physiological withdrawal and how much to a psychological compulsion to smoke is unknown. It does appear that some form of tolerance of nicotine may develop if the compound is regularly and repeatedly ingested. It may take progressively more and more nicotine to achieve the same level of central stimulation. Clinically, this would be manifested by an increase in the number of cigarettes that an individual smoked in a day.

Side Effects and Toxicity

In the CSN, side effects of nicotine usually consist of cortical stimulation, irritability, and tremors. Peripherally, side effects are usually manifested by intestinal cramps, diarrhea, increased heart rate and blood pressure, possible vomiting, and water retention.

The serious side effects of nicotine are many and indeed alarming when one considers the widespread use of this drug.

Cigarette smoking has now been demonstrated beyond reasonable doubt to induce serious chronic toxicity, although it is not clear whether it is the nicotine or some other ingredient of tobacco that is responsible for the toxicity.

It has been estimated that 360,000 persons die annually because of tobacco use and that one's life is shortened 14 minutes for every cigarette smoked. Smoking is thus the greatest public health hazard in the United States and the nation's most preventable cause of death.[12]

In the lungs, chronic smoking results in a smoker's syndrome characterized by difficulty in breathing, wheezing, chest pain, lung congestion, and increased susceptibility to infections of the respiratory tract. Cigarette smoking impairs ventilation and greatly increases the risk of emphysema (a form of irreversible lung damage).

In addition to this chronic bronchial irritation, there is a positive correlation between smoking and the incidence of lung cancer. Such cancers are caused, it is believed, by the tars and other chemicals in tobacco rather than by the nicotine. Studies demonstrate that for every nonsmoker who dies from lung cancer, 11 cigarette smokers will die from the same cause. Heavy use of tobacco is responsible for the fact that cancer of the lung is now the most common cancer among American men. In addition, cigarette smoking is also associated with a higher incidence of cancers of the oral cavity and esophagus.

Considerable interest has recently been focused on the effects of chronic tobacco smoking on the cardiovascular system. Cigarette smokers have a higher death rate from coronary heart disease than do nonsmokers. Since nicotine increases both heart rate and blood pressure, smokers respond with sustained increases in blood pressure, which increase the workload of the heart. There is now some evidence that cigarette smoke may increase the formation of blood clots.

In addition to its effects on the lungs, the heart, and the vasculature, cigarette smoking exerts a variety of other toxic effects that will not be elucidated here since it should be clear by now that the toxicity of nicotine (and cigarettes) is as high as that of any other psychoactive drug.

Effects in Pregnancy

There is now strong evidence that cigarette smoking affects the developing fetus. Cigarettes increase the rates of spontaneous abortion, stillbirths, and early postpartum death of infants. It appears that infants born of smoking mothers are at least twice as likely to be stillborn as infants born of nonsmoking mothers. There even appears to be a relationship between the number of cigarettes smoked per day and the percentage of stillbirths. There is evidence that infants born of nonsmoking mothers may be heavier than those born of smoking mothers, at least during the first year of life.

Thus, as has been so often stressed throughout this book, psychoactive drugs are readily distributed through the placenta and may exert potent effects on the developing fetus. Because nicotine is among the most commonly used psychoactive drugs in our society, the situation is even more serious. Thus, nicotine should be considered as being possibly deleterious to the fetus and therefore contraindicated during pregnancy. Since a woman often does not realize that she is pregnant until six, eight, or even more weeks have elapsed, it might be suggested that the drug is contraindicated for all women who might become pregnant. Further evidence has been gathered to indicate that smoking during the last six months of pregnancy results in a statistically significant increase in the numbers of stillbirths.

From the evidence we may conclude that, if we are interested in the effects of drugs on the fetus, on fetal development, and on newborn infants, nicotine should be classified as being contraindicated throughout the entire nine months of pregnancy and the duration of breast-feeding thereafter.

NOTES

1. For the historical development and background, see E. M. Brecher and *Consumer Reports* editors, *Licit and Illicit Drugs* (Mount Vernon, N.Y.: Consumers Union, 1972.

2. F. H. Meyers, E. Jawetz, and A. Goldfien, *Review of Medical Pharmacology,* 3d ed. (Los Altos, Calif.: Lange Medical Publications, 1972), p. 280.

3. *Interim Report of the Commission of Inquiry into the Non-medical Use of Drugs.* Gerald Le Dain, chairman (Ottawa: Information Canada, 1970), p. 52.

4. G. Smith and H. K. Beecher, "Amphetamine Sulfate and Athletic Performance," *Journal of the American Medical Association* 170 (1959): 542–47.

5. E. Jones, *Life and Work of Sigmund Freud,* vol. I (New York: Basic Books, 1961), pp. 82–83.

6. Brecher, *Licit and Illicit Drugs,* pp. 272–77.

7. *Ibid.,* pp. 302–7.

8. A. Goldstein, L. Aronow, and S. M. Kalman, *Principles of Drug Action* (New York: Harper & Row, 1968), p. 185.

9. *Ibid.,* pp. 647–53 and 663–68.

10. *Ibid.,* p. 733.

11. Brecher, *Licit and Illicit Drugs,* pp. 272–77 and 302–7.

12. R. L. Volle and G. B. Koelle, "Ganglionic Stimulating and Blocking Agents," In *Pharmacological Basis of Therapeutics,* 5th ed., L. S. Goodman and A. Gilman, eds. (New York: Macmillan, 1975), p. 569.

Chapter 6

The Opiates: Morphine and Other Narcotics

In this chapter, we will discuss the pharmacological, physiological, psychological, and behavioral effects induced by a group of compounds referred to as *opiates, narcotic analgesics, or strongly addictive analgesics*. The term *opiate* refers to any natural or synthetic drug that exerts actions upon the body similar to those induced by morphine, the major pain-relieving agent obtained from the opium poppy. The term *narcotic* has numerous meanings and usually is defined in widely varying terms by law-enforcement officers, lawyers, physicians, scientists, and laymen. Here, *narcotic* will be used to refer to those drugs that have both a sedative (sleep-inducing) and an analgesic (pain-relieving) action, a definition that restricts the term to the opiates.

The major medical uses of the opiates are for the relief of pain, the treatment of diarrhea, and the relief of coughing. Since the opiates are addictive (that is, are capable of inducing tolerance and physiological and psychological dependence), many synthetic drugs that are like morphine in action have been synthesized in attempts to duplicate the therapeutic usefulness of the opiates and avoid the addictive qualities of the opiates. With only one or two exceptions, these attempts to separate the analgesic effects from the euphoria-producing effects, which are those associated with compulsive abuse, have been unsuccessful.

HISTORICAL BACKGROUND

Opium occurs naturally and is obtained from the opium poppy, *Papaver somniferum*. The earliest descriptions of the psychological and physiological effects of opium appear to have been written in about 300 B.C., although references to opiates have been found dating to about 3000 B.C. Opium appears to have been used in early Egyptian, Greek, and Arabian cultures primarily for its constipating effect in the treatment of diarrhea. Later, opium's sleep-inducing properties were noted by Greek and Roman writers such as Homer, Virgil, and Ovid. Opium was frequently used by the Greeks to treat a variety of medical problems, including snake bite, asthma, cough, epilepsy, colic, urinary complaints, headache, and deafness. The Greeks also appeared to use the drug recreationally, and opium cakes and candies were commonly available on the streets. Addiction to opium was common, even among high-standing military and political figures of Rome.

From the early Greek and Roman days through the sixteenth and seventeenth centuries, the medicinal and recreational uses of opium were well established throughout Europe. Since much of the opium came from the Near East and the Orient, a bustling trade in opium existed between East and West. Indeed, control of opium was a central issue in the opium wars in China in 1839.

Through the centuries, from 3000 B.C. to A.D. 1800, the opiates used medicinally and recreationally consisted of the crude opium obtained from the opium poppy. Opium, however, is a resinous material that contains at least twenty different substances. It was not until the early 1800s that a chemist named Serturner isolated the primary active drug in opium, *morphine*. The development of morphine revolutionized the use of the opiates, and since then morphine (rather than crude opium) has been used throughout the world for the medical treatment of pain and diarrhea.

In the United States, morphine and opium are both widely used and have been since the nineteenth century. Until 1914, both drugs, for prescription and nonprescription use, were as accessible as aspirin is today, being freely available from physicians, drug stores, and general stores, by mail order, and in patent medicines sold through a variety of channels. It was not until after the Civil War (when opiate addiction was referred to as "soldier's disease") and the invention of the hypodermic needle in 1856 that a new type of drug user appeared in the United States; one who administered opiates to himself by injection. At about this time, there was a large influx of Chinese laborers who freely smoked opium.

By the early part of the twentieth century, opium use was widespread and it was estimated that one out of every 400 Americans was addicted to opium or one of its derivatives. Concern began to mount over the possible dangers of opiates and the dependence that they might induce. In 1914, the Harrison Narcotic Act was passed and the use of most opiate products was placed under strict controls. Nonmedical uses of opiates were banned. The history of the development of these controls and their effect on opiate use is fascinating. Brecher provides a lucid description of the changes in populations of addicts that were brought about by the Harrison Act and the various laws and decisions that followed it.[1]

The use of opiates is deeply entrenched in society, widespread, attractive, difficult to treat, and impossible to stop. The pharmacology of the opiates should be discussed in the same manner as that of any other class of psychoactive drugs that exert effects that can be pleasurable to the user, affect behavior, produce a pattern of tolerance and physiological dependence, and can potentially be compulsively misused. Emotional reactions or extensive legal efforts have failed, and will most likely continue to fail, to eradicate the recreational uses of these drugs. The opiates will continue to be used in medicine since, as pain-relieving agents, they are irreplaceable by other compounds. In addition, the profound effects of the opiates on the central nervous system induce an enormous liability for compulsive abuse, a liability that is likely to resist any efforts at total control.

CHEMISTRY

The term *opium* refers to the crude resinous exudate obtained from the opium poppy. Crude opium contains a wide variety of ingredients including *morphine* and *codeine*, both of which are widely used in medicine. The bulk of the ingredients of opium, however, consists of such organic substances as resins, oils, sugars, and proteins that account for more than 75 percent of the weight of the opium but exert little pharmacological activity. Morphine is the major pain-relieving drug found in opium, being approximately 10 percent of the crude exudate. Codeine is structurally closely related to morphine, although it is much less potent and amounts to only 0.5 percent of the opium extract. *Heroin* does not occur naturally but is a semisynthetic derivative produced by a chemical modification of morphine that increases the potency. It takes only 3 mg of heroin to produce the same analgesic effect as 10 mg of morphine (heroin being three times as potent as morphine). However, at equally effective doses (3 mg of heroin compared with 10 mg of morphine), it may be difficult to distinguish between the effects of the two compounds.

Several totally synthetic opiates are available. These are drugs that exert effects like those of opium but are synthetically produced in a laboratory. Meperidine (Demerol) and methadone (Dolophine) are both synthetic opiate narcotics. Meperidine is between 10 and 20 percent as potent as morphine (100 mg of meperidine being approximately equal in potency to between 10 and 20 mg of morphine). Methadone has approximately the same analgesic potency as morphine but induces less euphoria. Currently, methadone is being used in the treatment of opiate dependence.

MEDICAL USES

The primary medical uses of the opiates are for the relief of pain, the treatment of diarrhea, and the relief of cough, all disorders for which the opiates have been used since well before the sixteenth century. Despite intensive research, few other drugs have come even close to the opiate narcotics for use in the treatment of either pain or diarrhea. Although codeine is an extremely effective drug for the relief of cough, several newer synthetic compounds have been shown to be effective. In most nonprescription cough preparations, the codeine has been replaced by newer drugs such as dextromethorphan, a synthetic, nonnarcotic, nonanalgesic cough depressant with a very low potential for compulsive abuse. Nevertheless, morphine and related opiates will retain a vital and special place in the armamentarium of the physician as essential agents in the struggle against pain.

As the name *narcotic* implies, the opiates are capable of inducing sleep, but because of the euphoria they induce and because they are likely to be misused, they are seldom used medically for inducing sleep. However, where pain is present and sleep is necessary, the use of an opiate narcotic to supplement the sleep-inducing properties of a barbiturate is indicated. The barbiturates and other sedative-hypnotic compounds are not analgesic—that is, they do *not* relieve pain—and if pain is present, barbiturates may have little sedative or hypnotic effect.

ABSORPTION, DISTRIBUTION, METABOLISM, AND EXCRETION

The opiates (morphine and codeine) and their synthetic or semisynthetic equivalents (meperidine, heroin, and methadone) may be given by different routes. They may be administered orally, parenterally, or by inhalation. In general, absorption from the gastrointestinal route is slower and considerably less complete than absorption from either parenteral or inhalation routes. The opiate narcotics when given orally exist in the stomach in a fat-insoluble form that is only poorly absorbed from the stomach into the bloodstream. Absorption is delayed and occurs largely from the intestine. The blood level of drug that may be reached after a given oral dose of opiate is usually only half or less than that which may be achieved when the drug is administered by injection because absorption is incomplete. One of the few advantages of giving an opiate by mouth rather than by injection is that, because of this slow rate of absorption, the drug reaches the bloodstream slowly and is therefore metabolized at a slower rate, which may result in a somewhat longer duration of action in the body. In general, oral administration of an opiate results in erratic and unpredictable absorption when compared with administration of the drug by injection or by inhalation.

The opiates may be administered by intramuscular, subcutaneous, or intravenous injection; in nonmedical situations, the subcutaneous ("skin-popping") and intravenous ("main-lining") techniques are commonly used. The problems and limitations of the injection of drugs, delineated in Chapter 1, include accidental overdose, rapid onset of adverse drug reaction, necessity of sterile technique, and inability to recall the drug if too much is administered. The latter point may sometimes be circumvented, however, since specific pharmacological antagonists to opiates do exist, such as nalorphine (Nalline). This will be discussed later in this chapter.

As is well known from the history of opium smoking among Eastern cultures, the opiates may be administered by inhalation and absorbed through the lungs, either by sniffing the powdered drug or, more commonly, by inhalation of the smoke from burning crude opium. In either case, the opiates are rapidly and completely absorbed. In fact, the rapidity of onset of drug action rivals that of intravenous injection. (Refer back to Chapter 1 for a more complete discussion of the absorption of drugs from the lungs following inhalation.)

Opiates administered intravenously are not thought to have the immediate onset of psychoactive action of the barbiturates. It may take between 30 and 60 minutes to achieve significant levels of some opiates in the brain following intravenous injection, which indicates that the blood-brain barrier provides a significant impediment to the entry of opiates into the brain. The scientific demonstration of the slow penetration of opiates into the brain leaves unanswered the "rush" experienced by "main-liners" (individuals who inject opiates intravenously and who receive an immediate and intense pleasure seconds after the injection). It is not known whether the "rush" results from an action of the drug in the brain (it may get into the brain faster than scientists think) or from a powerful action on the peripheral nervous system or the cardiovascular system.

The opiates exist in the bloodstream in a fat-insoluble form. Since the blood-brain barrier is fairly impermeable to drugs in such form, the opiates only slowly penetrate the brain and only small amounts of some opiates ever reach the brain. Although the primary site of action of morphine, for example, is the CNS, only about 20 percent of the total amount of drug administered ever reaches brain tissue. In contrast, much heroin will pass the blood-brain barrier into the CNS, even though heroin and morphine have very similar structures; about 10 times as much heroin will reach the brain after injection of equal amounts of both drugs. Perhaps this may explain why the flash or rush with intravenous heroin is so much more intense than that perceived after injection of morphine. The opiates also reach all body tissues, including the fetus, and infants born of addicted mothers are physically dependent on opiates and may exhibit withdrawal symptoms unless they are given the drug.

Literally thousands of papers have been published in the scientific literature on the metabolism and excretion of morphine and the other opiates. In general, these studies have demonstrated that the opiates are largely metabolized by the liver before they are excreted by the kidneys. Small amounts of both codeine and heroin are metabolized by the body into morphine, which is further metabolized into inactive products that are finally excreted by the kidneys. Metabolism of most opiates is rapid; therefore, the durations of action of these drugs average four or five hours, a factor of considerable importance to the addict who must continually seek and administer the drug at intervals as short as three to five hours.

PHARMACOLOGICAL EFFECTS

Morphine and the other natural and synthetic opiates exert their major effects primarily on the central nervous system, the eye, and the gastrointestinal tract. In chronic morphine use or in acute morphine poisoning, a physiological syndrome consisting of sedation (which can lead to coma), chronic constipation, decreased respiratory rate, and pinpoint pupils is observed.

One of the prime medical uses of the opiates is in the relief of pain. The mechanism by which the opiate narcotics reduce pain is unknown. Very little is known about the physiology of pain or even the localization within the brain of areas where pain is felt or appreciated. Neurophysiologists even today have great difficulty in describing what pain is, where it is, or what modifies it. For example, our ignorance about the reasons why acupuncture may alleviate pain indicates our level of understanding of pain. Current research is slowly beginning to unravel some of the mysteries about pain and about which areas of the brain are affected by morphine. It now appears that morphine may have some specificity for norepinephrine, serotonin, and dopamine neurons (see Appendix II). Beyond this, however, we know very little about how morphine affects the brain or in what specific parts of the brain opiates act. Therefore, while we describe the actions of the opiates on their major target organs, the reader must remember that the precise mechanisms through which the drugs exert their effects have not been elucidated.

The Central Nervous System

Morphine exerts a narcotic action manifested by analgesia, drowsiness, changes in mood, and mental clouding.[2] The major medical action of morphine sought in the CNS is analgesia, which may usually be induced by doses below those that cause other effects on the CNS, such as sedation, respiratory depression, or vomiting. The mechanism of this analgesic action is unknown. What is known, however, is that relief of pain may occur in the absence of a depression of other senses: vision, hearing, touch, or pressure sense are not affected. In fact, this analgesic action does not appear to result from a decrease of pain impulses into the brain. What appears to happen is that, after the administration of the opiate, there is an altered perception of the painful stimulus; the pain is still present and felt, but does not bother the patient and it is not appreciated as being painful. Thus, it would appear that, rather than decreasing the stimulus of pain, these drugs decrease the suffering associated with the pain by altering the patient's awareness of it: the patient no longer cares that he or she hurts. Nonnarcotic analgesics, such as aspirin, are thought to decrease the pain impulses into the brain. More complete explanation of the analgesic actions of opiates must await identification of the mechanisms of pain within the brain, something that so far has eluded characterization.

A second major action of morphine and the other opiates on the CNS is to depress respiratory centers located in the brainstem. The result of this action is a marked decrease in the rate of respiration. At high doses of opiates, respiration may become so slow and irregular that life may be threatened. Indeed, the cardinal acute toxic effect of opiate narcotics is respiratory depression. This effect far outweighs all other adverse effects of this class of drugs. Death, when induced by opiates, is almost always secondary to failure of respiration.

In addition to this depressant action on respiration, opiates suppress the "cough center," which is also located in the brainstem. Such an action is thought to underlie the utility of opiate narcotics as cough suppressants. Codeine appears to be particularly effective in this action and is widely used for this purpose.

In contrast to these depressant actions on the braimstem, morphine also exerts a variety of *excitatory* effects. One such excitatory effect is a stimulation of the "vomiting center," resulting in nausea and vomiting, which are side effects frequently seen in patients to whom opiates are administered. Excitatory effects of morphine and other opiates on the cerebral cortex are quite complex. Cats, for example, are usually wildly excited following morphine administration; in humans the usual effect of morphine is sedative. Some people, however, are made excited and even maniacal by morphine. In addition, morphine is usually described as producing a state of euphoria, despite the fact that some individuals may experience a foggy sensation that is perceived as being unpleasant or dysphoric. Therefore, as one can appreciate, the mixed excitant and depressant effects of morphine on the CNS are complicated and the behavioral effects and the subjective experiences that follow morphine administration may vary markedly between individuals.

Morphine exerts EEG effects similar in many respects to those produced by the barbiturates. The EEG shifts from one characteristic of alertness to one characteristic of sleep or drowsiness. Also, like the barbiturates, morphine suppresses REM (dream) sleep and, with repeated administration, the EEG patterns return toward those characteristic of alertness; the EEG patterns observed in a tolerant individual differ from the EEG patterns seen in an individual who has no tolerance.

The Eye

A prominent physiological action of morphine is a decrease in the size of the pupil, producing pinpoint pupils by a mechanism that is not known but that originates in the brain rather than directly in the eye. Opiate overdose is often diagnosed by the observation of pinpoint pupils and a slow rate of respiration.

The Gastrointestinal Tract

The opiates have been used for centuries for the relief of diarrhea and for the treatment of dysentery, uses developed long before these agents were used as analgesics or euphoriants. The effects of the opiates on the gastrointestinal tract appear to be exerted both on the stomach and on the intestine. In the intestine, peristaltic movements (or waves), which normally propel food down the intestine, are markedly diminished, while the tone of the intestine is greatly increased to the point where almost complete spastic paralysis of movement occurs. This combination of decreased propulsion and increased tone leads to a marked decrease in the movement of food through the intestine. This stasis is followed by a dessication (drying) of the feces, which hardens the stool and further retards the advance of material through the intestine. All these effects contribute to the constipating properties of opiates. Indeed, no more effective drugs have been yet developed for the therapeutic treatment of severe diarrhea.

PSYCHOLOGICAL EFFECTS

Morphine produces analgesia, drowsiness, mood changes, and mental clouding.[3] In most people, opiates induce an extremely pleasant euphoric state, but such a reaction is not universal. On first use of an opiate, some individuals experience a dysphoria, consisting of anxiety and fear, lethargy, apathy, sedation, mental clouding, lack of concern, inability to concentrate, nausea, and vomiting. The effects of the opiate narcotics therefore vary considerably from person to person and may be influenced by the set and setting in which the drug is administered. Even if the first exposure to opiates results in dysphoria, repeated exposures usually result in a state of euphoria, consisting of warmth, a feeling of well-being, peacefulness, and contentment, accompanied by feelings of boundless energy and strength or, conversely, a pleasant dreamlike state, a turning inward, and sleep.

Regular users and those who are psychologically attracted to these drugs describe the effects of the intravenous injection of opiates in ecstatic and often in sexual terms. This euphoria induces a powerful compulsion to continue to use the drug. However, the euphoric effect becomes progressively *less* intense, and users then inject the drug for one or more of several possible reasons: in an attempt to reexperience the extreme euphoria of the first few injections, to maintain a state of pleasantness and well-being, to prevent mental discomfort associated with reality, or to prevent the physical discomforts associated with not injecting the drug.

Perhaps part of the psychological attraction to the opiates is related to their ability to alter the perception of pain by inducing a lack of concern for or indifference to the pain. Medical practitioners and researchers often tend to describe pain in physical terms: a person who has cancer or breaks a leg is in pain. However, we cannot discount the possibility of emotional or psychological pain to which no organic cause may be ascribed. Thus, in certain individuals who are attracted to the opiates, it is perhaps the ability of the opiates to dull an indeterminable psychological pain that may be partly responsible for the profound psychological effects and the feeling of well-being that the drug may induce.

TOLERANCE AND DEPENDENCE

Tolerance to morphine and to the other opiate narcotics varies with the particular physiological response, the dose, and the frequency of administration. With all opiates, tolerance to the respiratory depressant, analgesic, euphoric, and sedative effects develops, but not usually to the pupil-constricting or constipating effects.

The rate at which tolerance develops varies widely. With intermittent use of an opiate, little if any tolerance develops. When "sprees" of drug use are separated by prolonged drug-free periods, the opiates will retain their initial efficacy. For example, if a person uses opiates for recreational purposes only on weekends, low doses may continue to be effective and doses may not have to be markedly increased (unless, of course, a greater or more intense effect is desired). However, usually within a year, Saturday and Sunday "sprees" tend to begin on Friday night and go through Monday morning. Soon the drug is also used on Tuesday, Wednesday, and Thursday, and the "spree" is now a seven-day-week addiction.

As soon as this pattern of repeated administration occurs, tolerance develops and may become so marked that phenomenal doses have to be administered in order to maintain a state of euphoria or prevent discomfort. This tolerance appears to be due both to the induction of drug-metabolizing enzymes in the liver and to the adaptation of neurons in the brain to the presence of the drug, the tolerance developing within the brain being much greater than the tolerance in the liver.

In addition to the development of tolerance to one opiate, *cross-tolerance* develops, so that an individual who becomes tolerant to one opiate will also exhibit a tolerance to all other natural or synthetic opiates, even if they are chemically dissimilar. This cross tolerance is similar to that exhibited by various sedative-hypnotics (see Chapter 3). Cross tolerance, however, does *not* develop between the opiate narcotics and the sedative-hypnotics. An individual who has developed a tolerance to morphine will also be tolerant to heroin but not of alcohol or barbiturates. This latter point is extremely important, since accidental death may result from the additive effects of a sedative and an opiate. For example, if an individual takes moderate doses of opiates and then drinks alcohol or takes a sedative-hypnotic drug, additive depression of respiration will occur and could lead ultimately to coma and death. Deaths from the combined effects of opiates and general depressants are not at all uncommon.

In Chapter 1, we described *physical dependence* as a state in which people do not function properly without a drug. Physical dependence is characterized by the development of the symptom complex called *withdrawal* when the drug is not administered. Physical dependence on the sedative-hypnotic compounds is characterized by hyperexcitability when the drug is withheld. Withdrawal of the central stimulants such as amphetamine is followed by profound physical and emotional depression. Symptoms of withdrawal from the opiate narcotics are similar to a severe case of the flu; they last for four to seven days and are characterized by restlessness and craving for the drug, sweating, extreme anxiety, fever, chills, violent retching and vomiting, increased respiratory rate (panting), cramping, insomnia, explosive diarrhea, and nearly unbearable aches and pains. The magnitude of these withdrawal symptoms depends upon the dose and frequency of drug administration, the duration of drug dependence, and the opiate used. For example, withdrawal signs following the removal of methadone are usually less severe than those observed following the removal of heroin.

Withdrawal from the opiates also differs from withdrawal from the barbiturates in that, despite the fact that the effects are uncomfortable and seemingly unbearable, they are seldom life threatening. Convulsions leading to respiratory paralysis and death are not observed during withdrawal from an opiate.

Too often, extremely vivid accounts of the withdrawal symptoms are presented as part of the attempt to discourage the recreational use of heroin, opium, morphine, or other opiate narcotics. The dependence and withdrawal syndrome should not be held as the *only* reason that these drugs should not be used for recreational purposes. The opiates are extremely potent, valuable, and irreplaceable drugs for the treatment of pain. But they also have the capability of inducing a state of euphoria and relief from psychological pain, which may lead to a powerful compulsion to misuse them. In addition, intravenous injection of these drugs is capable of inducing a "rush" similar to that obtained from the amphetamines and which can only be described in ecstatic or sexual terms.

The opiates induce profound tolerance and physiological dependence, the consequences of which are important both medically and sociologically since the dependent and tolerant opiate user is difficult to treat and must frequently resort to crime to support the habit and reach a source of supply. Tolerance leads to the need for massive doses of drugs in order to prevent withdrawal, alleviate pain (physical or psychological), and maintain a state of euphoria. Drugs are extremely expensive when it becomes necessary to purchase them illegally, even though they may be inexpensive if it were possible to purchase them legitimately. It is not the tolerance and dependence that are so harmful as the lengths to which the individual is forced to go in order to procure adequate supplies of drugs. A person who has access to inexpensive, medical-quality narcotics and sterile needles and syringes supplied through legitimate sources is capable of leading a fairly normal life despite his tolerance to and physical dependence upon an opiate.

SYNTHETIC NARCOTIC ANALGESICS

The pharmacological effects of morphine (a naturally occurring opium alkaloid) and heroin (a semisynthetic derivative of morphine) have been presented above. Figure 6.1 presents the structural formulas of these two drugs together with those of four synthetically produced agents; these latter four are structurally unrelated to either morphine or heroin, but they have about the same qualitative pharmacological actions as morphine and differ from it only quantitatively. We will discuss these synthetic analgesics with reference to morphine and emphasize the differences.

Meperidine

Meperidine (Demerol) is a synthetic compound that was introduced into medicine in 1939. Although not originally studied as an analgesic, meperidine was soon discovered to have considerable analgesic activity. As Figure 6.1 shows, it is chemically quite dissimilar to morphine, and for many years meperidine was thought to be free of many of the undesirable properties associated with the use of opium alkaloids. It is now recognized that meperidine is addictive and will substitute for morphine or heroin in addicts. Meperidine is widely available commercially and is probably the narcotic most frequently abused by physicians and others within the medical profession. Because it is the narcotic analgesic most widely prescribed for pain relief in hospitalized patients, it is therefore an extremely commonly encountered agent in physician-induced addiction of patients.

Like those of morphine, the pharmacological effects of meperidine are characterized by analgesia, sedation, euphoria, and respiratory depression. One interesting difference is that meperidine does not cause pinpoint pupils, but the pupils tend to dilate. Unlike morphine, meperidine is quite well absorbed when taken orally. This drug is therefore frequently prescribed when an orally administered, potent analgesic is needed.

Given by injection (subcutaneous or intramuscular), meperidine has a rapid onset of action (within 10 minutes) but a dura-

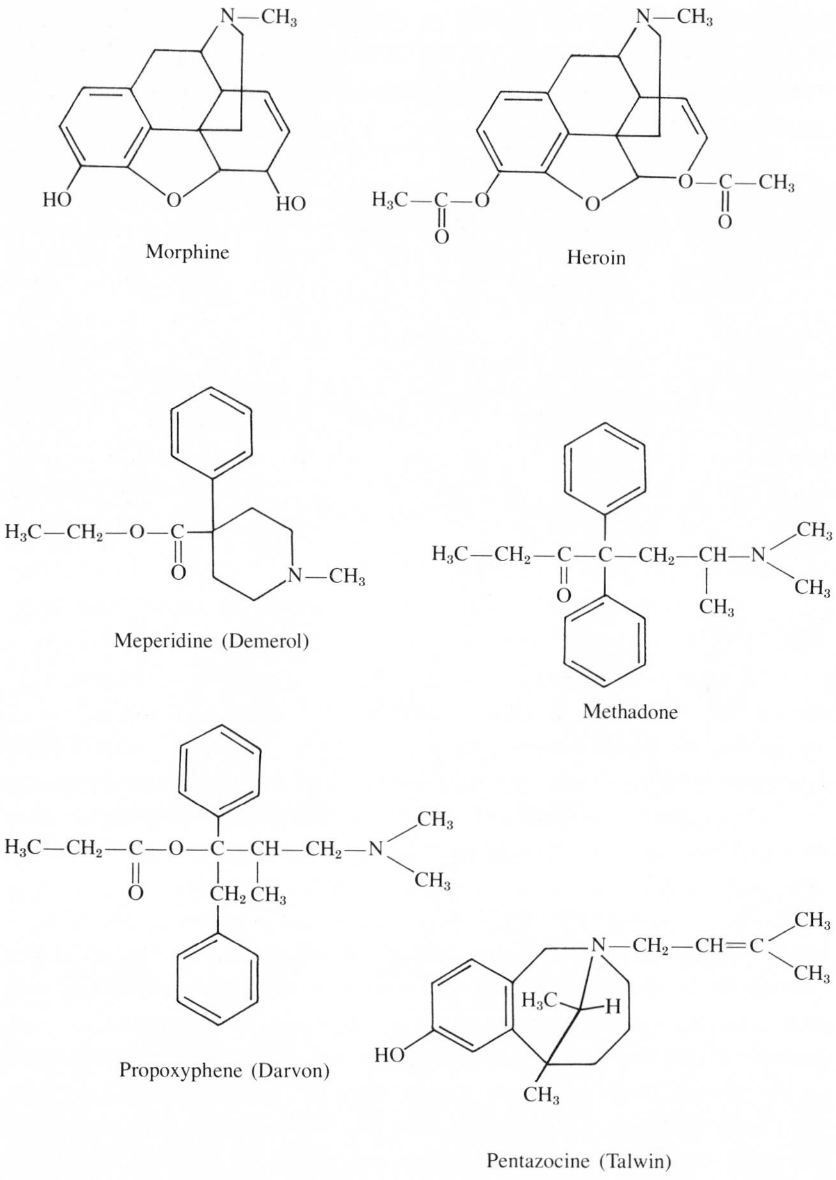

Morphine

Heroin

Meperidine (Demerol)

Methadone

Propoxyphene (Darvon)

Pentazocine (Talwin)

Figure 6.1. Structural formulas of morphine, heroin, and four synthetic narcotic analgesics.

tion of action that is considerably shorter than that of morphine (two to four hours). This short duration necessitates frequent reinjections for the relief of continuing pain. Unlike morphine, meperidine is not clinically useful for the treatment of cough or diarrhea.

Methadone

Methadone (Dolophine) is a synthetic opiate narcotic first synthesized by German chemists during World War II. The pharmacological activity of the drug is very similar to that of morphine. As stated by Jaffe and Martin, "The outstanding properties of methadone are its effective analgesic activity, its efficacy by the oral route, its extended duration of action in suppressing withdrawal symptoms in physically dependent individuals, and its tendency to show persistent effects with repeated administration."[4]

One of the most important current uses of methadone is in the controlled withdrawal of opiate addicts. In this situation, orally administered methadone is substituted for the injected opiate and the patient is then slowly withdrawn from methadone. The withdrawal is milder and less acute than that with morphine. Another important use is in methadone maintenance programs for opiate dependence. Since methadone is an effective agent when administered orally and since it has an extended duration of action, it is used as substitute therapy for other opiate narcotics. These uses of methadone are further discussed below.

Propoxyphene

Propoxyphene (Darvon) is an analgesic compound structurally very similar to methadone (Figure 6.1). As an analgesic its potency is somewhat less than that of codeine and approximately equal to that of therapeutic doses of aspirin. In large doses, opiate-like effects are seen, and when used intravenously, propoxyphene is recognized by addicts as a narcotic. Used orally, however, the abuse liability of propoxyphene is relatively low. Some cases of drug dependence have been reported, but to date they have not been of major concern. Abuse difficulties arise primarily when the drug is administered intravenously. Since commercial intravenous preparations are not available, such abuse is encountered only when individuals attempt to inject powder taken from the capsules intended for oral use.

Pentazocine

Pentazocine (Talwin) is a synthetic opiate analgesic compound that when administered orally has a potency comparable to that of codeine and when administered by injection has a potency approximately one-quarter that of morphine. The effects of pentazocine on the nervous system resemble those of morphine, including a significant depression of respiration.

In addition to these analgesic and respiratory-depressant activities, pentazocine administered to morphine- or heroin-dependent persons will only poorly substitute for these more potent agents and, indeed, the drug-dependent individual may experience withdrawal symptoms. Pentazocine may therefore be best considered as a low-potency opiate narcotic, which, because of low potency, will not totally substitute for more potent compounds.

ANTAGONISTS OF OPIATE NARCOTICS

In the above discussion, we noted that when pentazocine is administered to nonaddicts a morphinelike action was observed but when administered to morphine- or heroin-dependent individuals, the drug would not substitute and a withdrawal syndrome might be precipitated. This apparent contradiction in action can be explained by the fact that when pentazocine is administered to nonaddicted individuals the drug attaches to "opiate receptors" in the brain and produces the characteristic (although mild) narcotic actions of analgesia, sedation, euphoria, and respiratory depression. However, when pentazocine is administered to a person who is physically dependent on morphine, heroin, or another narcotic analgesic, the pentazocine competes with the more potent drug for these "opiate receptors," displacing much of the latter drug. In so doing, a drug that exerts a strong opiate action is displaced by one that exerts weaker activity. Therefore, whereas pentazocine is a narcotic when it is administered to normal individuals, it is a narcotic *antagonist* when it is administered to addicted persons. Such a drug with weak morphinelike activity in nonaddicts and a morphine-antagonist effect in addicted individuals is referred to as a *mixed agonist-antagonist*.

Nalorphine

The origin of a mixed agonist-antagonist occurred during the early 1950s, when it was demonstrated that *nalorphine* would precipitate an acute withdrawal syndrome in heroin addicts but was nevertheless an effective analgesic when administered to nonaddicts. The identification of a compound that was analgesic in nonaddicts yet did not substitute for heroin in addicts raised the hope that clinically useful compounds could be identified that would be free of abuse potential yet still have analgesic activity. Pentazocine (discussed above) is a recent development in the search for such a compound, and indeed this compound partly meets these objectives.

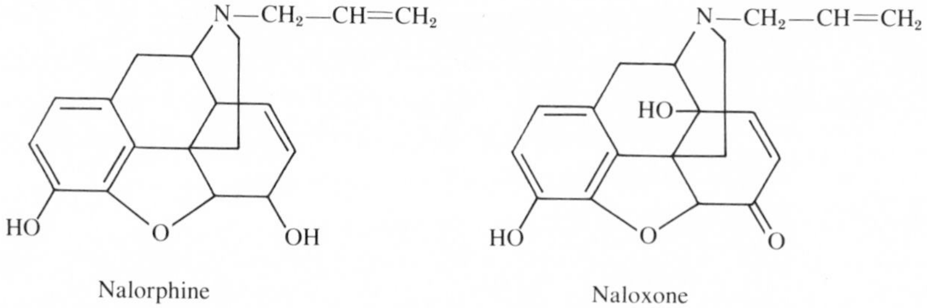

Figure 6.2. Structural formulas of two morphine antagonists.

Nalorphine (Figure 6.2) is structurally related to both morphine and heroin as well as to pentazocine. Administered to nondependent individuals, nalorphine is an effective analgesic. However, the drug produces dysphoria (rather than euphoria), leading to a range of unpleasant mental effects, including malaise, confusion, disorientation, and hallucinations. These effects limit its analgesic usefulness. Administered to an opiate-dependent person, nalorphine rapidly precipitates an acute withdrawal syndrome. At present, since nalorphine rapidly reverses the respiratory depression induced by morphine and heroin, it is clinically used to treat acute narcotic intoxication (overdoses). It is also used to reverse opiate-induced respiratory depression in newborns of mothers who have received narcotic analgesics.

Naloxone

Subsequent to the development of nalorphine, *naloxone* (see Figure 6.2) was synthesized. This drug differs from nalorphine in that it is almost devoid of morphinelike effects in normal persons. It is not analgesic, produces no euphoria, and does not depress respiration. However, naloxone is approximately seven times as potent as nalorphine in precipitating the withdrawal syndrome, and it retains this ability even when administered chronically. Naloxone is therefore referred to as a *pure narcotic antagonist*, since it is devoid of agonistic (morphinelike) effects and therefore is not subject to abuse.

The uses of naloxone are similar to those of nalorphine listed above. In the treatment of chronic narcotic dependence, addicts undergo drug withdrawal on a voluntary basis and are then administered daily doses of naloxone to prevent any euphoric effect if they should take subsequent doses of heroin or morphine. The utility of naloxone in such programs is limited by a short duration of action and the necessity of a parenteral route of administration (the drug is poorly absorbed orally). Currently being evaluated are new narcotic antogonists that may be orally administered and that have long durations of action. However, as we will discuss below, the effectiveness of using narcotic antagonists as a therapeutic approach to narcotic dependence has not been fully evaluated, and extensive clinical trials over several years will be necessary to determine long-term efficacy.

OPIATE NARCOTICS AND CRIME

The relationship between the use of opiates and the occurrence of crime is complex and charged with emotion. Blum and his associates stated that "no known drug, by itself, can be shown to 'cause' crime, although when the use of a drug is illegal, the 'crime' clearly rests upon the person's decision to acquire, possess, or use the drug illicitly."[5] If the use of a drug is defined as a crime, drug use *must* lead to crime. Laws have been passed to control the manufacture, distribution, and sale of opiates and many other psychoactive drugs, so that in the mere possession, use, or selling of any drug illegally a crime is necessarily committed.

Other factors in the relation of opiates and crime are perhaps more serious. For example, the illegal procurement of opiates is extremely expensive. A well-developed heroin habit may require the expenditure of anywhere from $20 to $150 a day. The same quantity of drug obtained legally would cost only a few cents. Obviously, there are very few legitimate ways in which most people may earn this amount of extra money. The individual has one of two choices: either to stop taking the drug, lose the euphoria, and go through withdrawal, or else to attempt to meet the necessary expenditure by turning to illegal activities, such as petty crimes, shoplifting, prostitution, and other, usually nonviolent, activities. The present laws seem to encourage crime. By making these drugs illegal, by making the addict a criminal, and by restricting trade by incarcerating the small-volume dealer (which forces prices upward), the laws force an individual to commit crimes in order to obtain his or her drug supply.

There is little evidence to indicate that crimes of violence are a direct consequence of the use of opiate narcotics. Individuals on opiates are usually quiet, passive, and seldom prone to violence. Still, while there is no evidence that opiates are a *cause* of violent crime, there is little doubt that among those addicts with a background of delinquency, the use of opiates is part of their total social activity, which includes crime. The use of opiates by these individuals may encourage or perpetuate associations in social or antisocial groups that may pose problems for the community and for society.

An important footnote must be added: Within the last few years there has been a drastic change in the pattern of the use of illicit drugs in our society. Whereas most opiate use was formerly confined to antisocial elements in our society, the use of opiates and other psychoactive drugs has spread into the suburbs and permeated all facets of community life. This tends to weaken even further the association between drugs and crime because now many users have sufficient funds to acquire necessary quantities of drugs. This new generation of drug users often does not use drugs continuously and thus may not develop tolerance or physical dependence. They use opiates, at least initially, only on "sprees" (for recreation) and do not need to buy large quantities of drugs. The fact that a person is an addict does not mean that he or she is a degenerate criminal or shabby, ill-shod, or malnourished. An individual tolerant to and dependent upon an opiate who is socially or financially capable of obtaining an adequate supply of good quality drug, sterile syringes and needles, and other paraphernalia may maintain his or her proper social and occupational functions, remain in fairly good health, and suffer little serious incapacitation as a result of the dependence.

TREATMENT OF THE OPIATE USER

The precise motivations for a person's becoming dependent upon opiate narcotics are far from clear. In the United States, there are two basic patterns of opiate use and dependence, as described by Jaffe:

> One involves individuals whose drug use begins in the context of medical treatment and who obtain the initial supplies through medical channels. This group constitutes a very small percentage of the addicted population. The other pattern begins with experimental or "recreational" drug use, progresses to more intensive use, and involves adolescents and young adults, with males far outnumbering females.[6]

The analgesia and euphoria induced by opiate narcotics is an attraction to their use. However, additional contributions to the incidence of opiate dependence appear to be sociological or psychological, rather than necessarily the result of a physiological or organic deficit in the individual. For example, in 1971, with the wide availability of opium and heroin in the Far East, about 45 percent of U.S. Army enlisted men in Vietnam had used opiates at least once.[7] About half of these users reported that at some time during their tour of duty in Vietnam they were physically dependent. It is unlikely that in this large number of young men there was a consistent organic deficit. Rather, the ready availability of opiates and the traumatic situation in which the soldiers were involved predisposed them to the use of these agents. It can therefore be seen that before any attempt is made to withdraw an addict permanently from opiate use, his or her underlying motivation for seeking the drug's positive reinforcement or reward (the euphoria, sedation, and analgesia) must be determined. In recent years, it has become clear that treatment and rehabilitation of .opiate users cannot reside *solely* in attempts to withdraw them from the drug but must include withdrawal from the positive reinforcements or life situations that were associated with opiate use. As Jaffe states:

> The indications for treatment vary with the drugs being used as well as with the social and cultural factors determining the particular pattern of drug use. Some patterns of drug use, such as the "recreational" use of marihuana, do not require treatment any more than does the occasional smoking of tobacco or the social use of alcohol. Such casual use is not without hazard, but this does not imply a treatable disorder. It is likely that changing views about drug use will continue to create grey areas where the indications for treatment are unclear. However, there is general agreement that treatment is appropriate for the adverse consequences of drug use and for the compulsive drug user who voluntarily seeks help.[8]

Until recent years, few thought a person who had become addicted to an opiate and who had used heroin intravenously could ever be satisfactorily rehabilitated and maintained in a functional, drug-free state, and addicts were routinely sentenced to imprisonment. Statistics indicate that such periods of imprisonment were not an effective deterrent or sufficient rehabilitation for the addict. At least 90 percent of those incarcerated for opiate use relapsed within six months of their release.

We have recently entered a more enlightened time in that we have recognized that to be an addict is to be ill and not necessarily criminal (recall the discussion of alcoholism). We handle the treatment and rehabilitation of the narcotic addict with a more positive, medically oriented approach. No longer do all physicians adhere to the concept that drug withdrawal must be the first step in treatment or that effective rehabilitation requires a carefully controlled, drug-free environment. The latter concept of rehabilitation started with the development of residential communities such as the Synanon Foundation in California, which undertake by social programs of group living and community involvement to assist former addicts in facing their problems, learning to understand themselves, and altering their behavior and life-styles. Such programs are effective. One frequently raised objection, however, is that addicts do not adjust to living in the "real world," because they are so completely involved in the small communal group. In addition, these programs are expensive and not capable of handling large numbers of drug-dependent individuals—an important point, since more and more persons within our society are using opiates.

These difficulties have led to the development of new programs designed to withdraw addicts, while they remain functioning members of their own communities, on oral doses of narcotic so that they need not purchase drugs on the black market. By so doing, the dependence on the needle, the subcultural involvement, and criminal orientation are decreased. It would be possible, of course, to continue to give patients the drugs they were using (heroin, morphine, and so on) and either maintain them on that dose (provided by a legitimate source) or else simply reduce the dose over a period of several days. However, as we mentioned above, methadone is an effective drug administered orally for suppressing withdrawal symptoms. Methadone can be substituted for any of the opiate analgesics currently available.

With *methadone substitution,* the opiate originally used (usually injected) is replaced by orally administered methadone. The dose of methadone is then slowly reduced over a period of 10 to 14 days. The withdrawal symptoms are rarely worse than those of a moderate "flulike" syndrome. The dose of methadone employed varies with the health of the patient and the amount of drug formerly used. With *methadone maintenance,* addicts are stabilized on methadone and, it is postulated, remain productive members of their communities so that it may not be necessary to withdraw the methadone. More recently, however, it has been found that after a period of stabilization (six months to two years) many former heroin addicts maintained on methadone can be gradually withdrawn from this drug over a period of several weeks. The withdrawal discomforts are relatively minor and some patients are able to complete the withdrawal processes and not relapse to the use of heroin, morphine, or other opiate. Others have completed the withdrawal but have later returned to heroin. Still other patients have discontinued withdrawal and have remained on methadone maintenance.

Methadone-substitution and methadone-maintenance programs have now been in operation for several years, and studies have concluded that methadone is an effective aid in the treatment of heroin addiction. It is also becoming clear that the methadone must be combined with intensive psychological counseling and adoption of a productive life-style. It is not enough merely to switch addicts from heroin to methadone and return them to the street. Indeed, this has happened in some programs and the result is often compulsive abuse of methadone or return to the use of heroin. Alternatives must be provided to the life-styles of the addicts and positive reinforcements introduced to replace the use of opiates before addicts will be successfully adjusted. Once these reinforcements are found outside the use of drugs, consideration can be given to discontinuing the methadone. Too rapid removal of methadone should be carefully avoided, however, since it may be more socially acceptable to maintain an individual on methadone than to return him or her to the street and to former habits of drug acquisition and use.

NOTES

1. E. M. Brecher and *Consumer Reports* editors, *Licit and Illicit Drugs* (Mt. Vernon, N.Y.: Consumers Union, 1972), pp. 47–100.

2. J. H. Jaffe and W. R. Martin, "Narcotic Analgesics and Antagonists," in *The Pharmacological Basis of Therapeutics,* 5th ed., L. S. Goodman and A. Gilman, eds. (New York: Macmillan, 1975), p. 247.

3. *Ibid.,* p. 247.

4. *Ibid.,* p. 268.

5. R. H. Blum and Associates, *Society and Drugs,* vol. 1 (San Francisco: Jossey-Bass, 1969), p. 290.

6. J. H. Jaffe, "Drug Addiction and Drug Abuse," in *The Pharmacological Basis of Therapeutics,* 5th ed., L. S. Goodman and A. Gilman, eds. (New York: Macmillan, 1975), p. 293.

7. L. Robins, *The Vietnam Drug User Returns: Final Report, Sept. 1973.* Special Action Office Monograph, Ser. A, no. 2 (Washington, D.C.: U.S. Government Printing Office, 1974).

8. Jaffe, "Drug Addiction and Drug Abuse," p. 312.

Chapter 7

Antipsychotic Tranquilizers: Drugs for Treating Schizophrenia and Other Psychoses

No one class of psychoactive drugs is effective in all mental disorders. Therefore such mental states as anxiety, neurosis, psychosis, schizophrenia, mania, and depression must be carefully differentiated.

Anxiety is a commonly used term referring to an unpleasant state of tension and uneasiness not usually associated with any specific stimulus.

Neurosis is similar and involves some degree of emotional disability, usually accompanied by anxiety. Neurotics have difficulty dealing with the common frustrations of life, with accepting themselves, and they are frequently troubled by chronic feelings of guilt.

Mania in its broadest sense refers to abnormal, uncontrollable, and possibly dangerous behavior. More commonly, mania is considered to be the excited phase of a mental disorder referred to as *manic-depressive psychosis. Depression* refers to a state of sadness, hopelessness, pessimism, and uselessness that can be so severe as to lead to impairment of function. Depression often occurs cyclically with mania, so that prolonged periods of manic behavior alternate with prolonged periods of depression.

Schizophrenia literally means "splitting of the mind" and refers to an inappropriateness or imbalance between the emotional reactions and the thought content associated with the emotions (that is, a split in the mind between emotions and mentation). Schizophrenia is characterized by disturbances in thinking, mood, and behavior. The thought disturbances include a distortion of reality, delusions, and hallucinations (usually auditory). The mood and behavioral disorders consist of ambivalence, apathy, withdrawal, and bizarre activity. The incidence of schizophrenia is estimated as 0.5 to 1 percent of the general population. Indeed, schizophrenics occupy approximately two-thirds of beds in mental hospitals and more than one-quarter of all hospital beds.

Psychosis is a general term referring to any mental disorder in which a person's mental capacity to recognize reality, communicate, and associate with others is impaired enough to interfere with his or her ability to deal with the ordinary demands of life. The psychoses are often subdivided into two major subclassifications according to their origin: (1) psychoses associated with a "brain syndrome" (a loss of nerve-cell function) such as would occur in drug-intoxication or dementia (see Chapter 3), and (2) those to which no organic cause has yet been found (such as schizophrenia).

MINOR VERSUS MAJOR TRANQUILIZERS

Many of the sedative-hypnotic drugs discussed in Chapter 3 are useful in treatment of anxiety states and neurotic behavior. They are not clinically useful in the management of schizophrenia or manic-depressive psychosis. They can not be relied upon to calm a psychotic patient without inducing pronounced depression of behavior or even deep sleep or anesthesia. The clinical antidepressants (Chapter 5) are useful in the treatment of some forms of depression but are of little value in the treatment of psychosis. In contrast, the antipsychotic tranquilizers have the ability to calm psychotic states and make the psychotic patient more manageable.

The "minor tranquilizers" discussed in Chapter 3 as being low-potency sedative-hypnotic compounds—chlordiazepoxide (Librium), diazepam (Valium), or meprobamate (Equanil)—differ from the drugs classified as "major tranquilizers" or, more correctly, "antipsychotic tranquilizers." A minor tranquilizer is a sedative-hypnotic compound useful in the treatment of anxiety and neurosis. A major or antipsychotic tranquilizer is a drug capable of relieving symptoms of psychosis (usually schizophrenia) and inducing a behavioral state characterized by psychomotor slowing, emotional quieting, and an indifference to external stimuli.

It is also important to note that the word *tranquilizer* implies the induction of a tranquil, calm, or pleasant state. This may indeed be true in the case of the minor tranquilizers since, as discussed in Chapter 3, sedative-hypnotic compounds can, in low doses, induce a state of disinhibition, euphoria, and relief from anxiety. In contrast, the psychological effects induced by the antipsychotic (or major) tranquilizers are seldom pleasant, seldom euphoric, and may be unpleasant or dysphoric when administered to individuals who are not psychotic. Hence, these agents are seldom encountered as drugs of abuse. Their importance in medicine, however, is well established. In addition, these agents have contributed in the laboratory to our knowledge of the physiological and biochemical bases of behavior and of mental disease.

HISTORICAL BACKGROUND

Clinical descriptions of psychotic patients (especially schizophrenics) date back to at least 1400 B.C. However, the isolation of these patients was the only known therapy until the early twentieth century. The concept of caring for individuals with mental disorders, rather than simply keeping them, did not become entrenched until the eighteenth century. Shock treatment in the eighteenth and nineteenth centuries consisted of twirling patients on a stool until they lost consciousness or dropping them through a trap door into an icy lake.

The only alternative to such drastic therapy was moral treatment, consisting of individualized attention, which today would resemble group and social therapy. Such treatment was probably an effective therapeutic approach to schizophrenic patients. However, with the introduction of huge mental hospitals, in which the personal approach disappeared, moral treatment and the therapeutic gains by such individualized attention were lost.

This therapeutic vacuum persisted until the mid-1930s, when Sakel introduced insulin coma as a therapeutic treatment. In this method, insulin was injected until the patient became hypoglycemic enough to lose consciousness and lapse into coma. Several such treatments were reported to aid schizophrenic behavior. Shortly thereafter, electroconvulsive therapy was introduced. In this technique, electrodes were placed on the patient's head and a current was applied until the patient had a seizure. A series of such seizure treatments was frequently effective in relieving the acute psychotic episode.

Prior to 1950, effective drugs for the treatment of psychotic patients were virtually nonexistent. Psychotic patients were usually permanently hospitalized. Between the end of World War II and the mid-fifties, more and more patients were residing in mental hospitals because more facilities were available, funds for the support and care of psychotic patients were increased, and there was more concern for the protection of other members in the community from psychotic patients. By 1955, there were over one-half million people in the United States residing in the state and local mental hospitals.

As can be seen from Figure 7.1, however, in 1955 there began a dramatic and steady reversal in this trend. By 1970 there were less

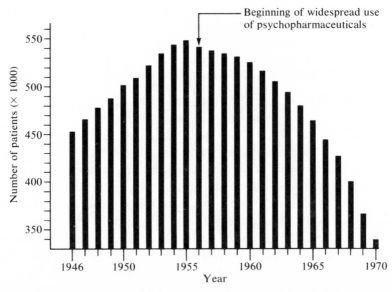

Figure 7.1. Numbers of resident patients in state and local government mental hospitals in the United States from 1946 through 1970. Note the dramatic change in the total population of mental hospitals that began in 1956 with the introduction into therapy of psychoactive drugs. [From V. C. Longo, *Neuropharmacology and Behavior* (San Francisco: W. H. Freeman, Copyright © 1972), fig. 1.3, p. 11. Modified from D. H. Efron, ed., *Psychopharmacology: A Review of Progress* (Washington, D.C.: U.S. Department of Health, Education, and Welfare, 1968).]

than 340,000 institutionalized patients. This decline in the number of residents in mental hospitals has occurred despite dramatic *increases* in the numbers of *admissions* to state hospitals. Indeed, between 1955 and 1965, the yearly rate of admissions almost doubled. The crucial factor has been that psychotic patients are now spending only one-quarter to one-third as long in hospitals as they were in 1955. Much of the change has been brought about since the introduction of new drugs effective in the management of psychotic behavior. Since these drugs have played such an important role within our society, a brief look at their historical development may be in order.

Although the prototype of the largest class of antipsychotic drugs (the phenothiazines) was synthesized in the late 1800s, it was not until approximately 1950 in France that a derivative of phenothiazine called promethazine (Phenergan) was found to have a strong sedative effect. In 1952, the French surgeon Laborit introduced the drug as an agent to deepen anesthesia induced by barbiturates. Later in 1952, researchers in a French pharmaceutical company developed another phenothiazine derivative, chlorpromazine (Thorazine), and included it in a "cocktail" administered to patients the night before surgery to allay their fears and anxieties. Chlorpromazine was then found to lower the amount of anesthetic drugs needed without itself inducing loss of consciousness, for it appeared to alter profoundly the patient's mental awareness. Thus, chloropromazine appeared to be distinct from the barbiturates and the other sedative-hypnotic drugs. Patients who had received chlorpromazine were quiet, conscious, sedated, and quite uninterested in and unconcerned about what was going on about them. Because of these effects, chlorpromazine was tried in the treatment of mental illness and was found to ameliorate psychotic episodes. Thus, for the first time, a drug had been found that specifically altered the manifestations of the psychotic process itself.

Chlorpromazine was introduced into the United States in 1954 and released for marketing in 1955. Its rapid success in the treatment of institutionalized psychotic patients is clearly seen in Figure 7.1.

At approximately the same time that chlorpromazine was introduced into the United States, another antipsychotic agent, unrelated to phenothiazine, was discovered and introduced into therapy. This compound was a drug called reserpine (Serpasil). If reserpine had been introduced and the phenothiazines not discovered, reserpine itself would have been the drug of choice for the treatment of psychotic patients, despite the fact that reserpine produces a number of bothersome side effects. Thus, since both drugs were introduced almost simultaneously, and both drugs were effective, the drug that produced fewer side effects was the one more widely used.

More recently, there have been attempts to identify antipsychotic drugs that might be superior to chlorpromazine and the other phenothiazines. One such class of drugs is the butyrophenones developed in Belgium in the mid-sixties. These compounds are structurally unrelated to the phenothiazines, but their pharmacological actions are similar. One of the butyrophenones, haloperidol (Haldol), has been marketed in the United States. This compound seems to have few significant advantages over the phenothiazines but is occasionally used for patients intolerant of phenothiazines.

THREE BIOLOGICAL THEORIES OF SCHIZOPHRENIA

As mentioned, two broad categories of psychotic states exist —those which can be explained by a loss of neurons in the brain and those for which no organic basis has been identified. Of the latter psychoses, two subcategories have been described: (1) manic-depressive psychoses and (2) schizophrenia. The norepinephrine theory of mania and depression was discussed earlier (early in Chapter 5). Here we will focus on current theories of the biological basis of schizophrenia. Two recent reviews of this topic have been published.[1,2]

The Altered Amine Theory

The *altered amine* hypothesis of schizophrenia is a theory based upon evidence that some schizophrenics excrete in their urine abnormal products of amine metabolism which are not found in the urine of normal patients. These altered substances are presumed to be methylated metabolites of dopamine, a normal transmitter within the central nervous system (see Appendix II). The relationship of these methylated metabolites of dopamine to schizophrenia is based in part upon the fact that some methylated products of normally occurring amines are hallucinogenic (see Chapter 8, the section on "Psychedelics Acting on Norepinephrine Neurons"). For example, mescaline is a methylated derivative of dopamine and norepinephrine and can induce a state resembling psychosis. It is not yet clear, however, whether this mescaline-induced psychosis is related to schizophrenia or, indeed, if schizophrenics have a common methylated amine that underlies the disorder.

The Dopamine Theory

A *dopamine* theory of schizophrenia is based upon pharmacological evidence that drugs that block dopamine receptors (see Appendix II) within the CNS are clinically useful in the treatment of schizophrenia. The phenothiazines, of which chlorpromazine is an example, are a class of drugs that block these dopamine receptors and that are currently the drugs of choice in the treatment of schizophrenia. Conversely, drugs that stimulate these dopamine receptors produce a state that closely resembles schizophrenia. Amphetamine (Chapter 5) is a drug that is a stimulant of dopamine (and NE) receptors, and amphetamine-induced psychosis is at the present time the best available model of acute schizophrenia. Klawans et al. have proposed that the physiological basis of schizophrenia is an increased sensitivity of dopamine receptors within the brain to the normal amounts of dopamine that are present.[3]

The Inherited Gene Theory

A third theory of schizophrenia is that this disease is a specific *inherited* disease resulting from a single mutant inherited gene. It has been hypothesized that there is as yet an undiscovered metabolic error that leads to the schizophrenic illness. Evidence in favor of this theory is based upon the fact that while the incidence of schizophrenia in the general population is approximately 1 percent, this increases to 7 to 16 percent in children with one schizophrenic parent and 40 to 68 percent if both parents are schizophrenic. No specific genetic deficit has yet been identified.

PHENOTHIAZINE DERIVATIVES

The phenothiazine derivatives are the most widely used drugs for the treatment of psychoses. These compounds are also widely used in the treatment of nausea and vomiting, for preanesthetic sedation, to delay ejaculation, and for relief from severe itching.

At present there are more than 20 phenothiazine derivatives available for clinical use. Our present discussion will center on the prototype agent of this class, chlorpromazine (Thorazine). Chlorpromazine is the most widely known and the most studied of the phenothiazine derivatives. Figure 7.2 shows the chemical structure of chlorpromazine together with the structures of reserpine and haloperidol, which are also used in the treatment of psychoses. The mechanism underlying the antipsychotic action of chlorpromazine and

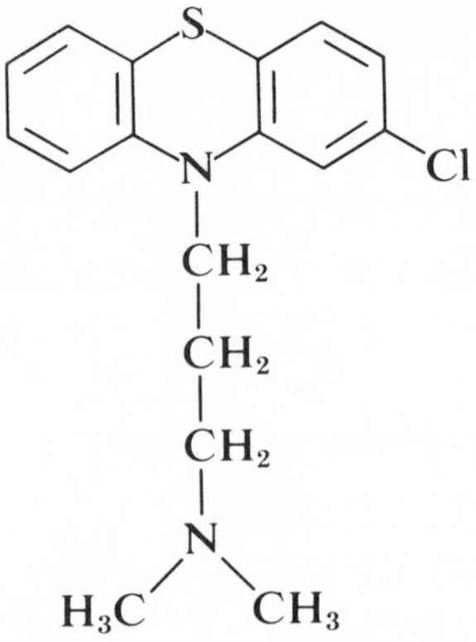

Chlorpromazine (Thorazine)

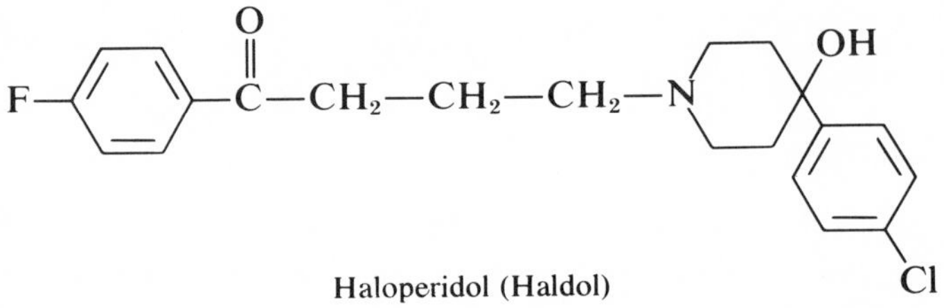

Haloperidol (Haldol)

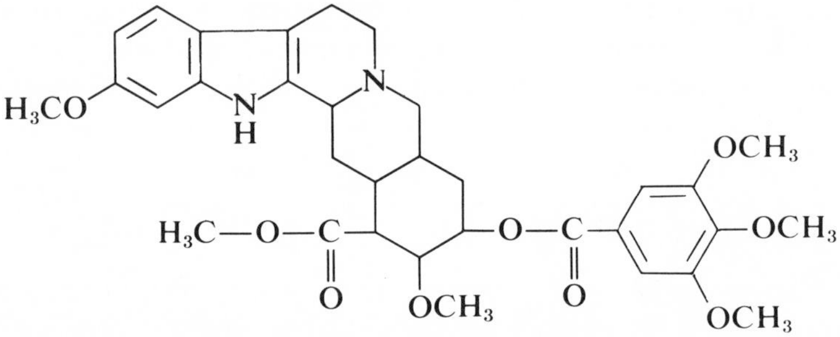

Reserpine (Serpasil)

Figure 7.2. Structural formulas of three representative antipsychotic tranquilizers. Chlorpromazine is a representative of the group of phenothiazine tranquilizers; about 20 other phenothiazine derivatives are available.

other phenothiazines is not entirely understood, although the effects of these agents can be accounted for by a blockade of dopamine receptors in various locations within the brain. Within the various subdivisions of the brain (see Appendix III) it can be noted that dopamine receptors occur most prominently in the reticular formation of the brainstem, the hypothalamus, the limbic system, and the basal ganglia. Examination of the consequences of blocking dopamine receptors in each of these structures will serve to explain the physiological and psychological effects of these drugs.

Absorption, Distribution, Metabolism, and Excretion

Although the phenothiazines are effectively absorbed from the gastrointestinal tract, such absorption is slow and incomplete. However, since a patient usually takes these drugs for long periods of time (even for a lifetime), the oral route of drug administration is still effective and is commonly used. Once in the bloodstream, the phenothiazines are rapidly distributed throughout the body. The levels of phenothiazines in the brain are low compared with the levels of phenothiazines found in other body tissues, the highest concentrations being found in the lungs, liver, adrenal glands, and spleen.

The metabolism and excretion of the phenothiazines is complex and among the slowest of any group of drugs. More than 160 metabolites of chlorpromazine have been postulated, and they appear to persist in the body for extremely long periods of time before they are excreted. It is not unusual for phenothiazine metabolites to be found in the urine a year or more after cessation of the administration of the drug. Even some unmetabolized phenothiazines may be present in the body a year after the drug is discontinued.

Pharmacological Effects

The phenothiazines produce dry mouth, dilated pupils, and blurred vision. Constipation, retention of urine, and increased heart rate may also be observed. There may be dilation of blood vessels, with resulting decreases in blood pressure, especially when an individual rises from a reclining position. The phenothiazines also affect certain hormones; they may disturb the menstrual cycle or block menstruation completely. They may induce lactation in women who are not pregnant.

In the central nervous system, which is the primary site of antipsychotic action, phenothiazines induce a syndrome characterized by psychomotor slowing, indifference to sensory stimuli, emotional quieting, and reduction of initiative. These effects are thought to be due to drug-induced blockade of dopamine receptors in the limbic system. As is discussed in Appendix III, the limbic system is involved in the regulation of emotion and emotional expression. Such suppression of limbic system activity appears to account for the emotional quieting and the calming effects induced by these drugs.

Through actions on the brainstem, the phenothiazines suppress certain centers involved both in behavioral arousal and in vomiting. By suppressing activity in the reticular formation, the phenothiazines induce an indifference to external stimuli such that greater levels of sensory input are necessary in order to alert or arouse an individual. In another area of the brainstem (the vomiting center), the phenothiazines block additional dopamine receptors and thereby inhibit vomiting. Indeed, these drugs are among the best antivomiting agents available.

It is also important to note that the phenothiazines exert prominent effects on an area of the brain referred to as the basal ganglia. Dopamine is an important neurotransmitter in this area, and, when absent, the result is expressed as Parkinson's disease. Replacing the absent dopamine (through the use of l-dopa) is an accepted treatment for this disease. Considering that the phenothiazines are dopamine blockers, it is logical to postulate that such blockade would have the same effect as depriving the individual of the transmitter itself; that is, the production of a Parkinsonianlike syndrome. Indeed, such is the case. Parkinsonian movements, including dulled expressions of the face, rigidity and tremor of the limbs, and slow movements are prominent side effects frequently associated with the use of antipsychotic drugs. In addition, it is now becoming increasingly evident that some of these drug-induced movement disorders may persist for prolonged periods after the drug is discontinued.

As discussed in Appendix III, the hypothalamus is intimately involved in emotional, eating and drinking, and sexual behavior and in control over the secretion of some hormones. By suppressing the function of the hypothalamus (again, by blocking dopamine receptors), phenothiazines interrupt these functions. By suppressing the appetite, food intake may be reduced. Sexually, the individual is difficult to arouse. In the male, ejaculation may be blocked. In the female, libido may be decreased, and there may be a blockade of ovulation, with suppression of normal menstrual cycles resulting in infertility. Breast enlargement may occur in the male, and females may begin spontaneously to secrete fluid from the nipples. Temperature-regulating centers in the hypothalamus are suppressed, and body temperature will fall in a cold room and rise in a hot room. Occasionally, large doses of phenothiazines may precipitate convulsions, and epileptic patients may have to increase their doses of antiepileptic drug in order to counteract this action. The frequency and severity of the side effects induced by the different phenothiazine derivatives vary, but, in general, all must be tolerated to some extent by the patient.

Psychological Effects

In general, chlorpromazine improves the mood and behavior of psychotic patients by producing an indifference to external stimuli and a reduction of initiative and anxiety without inducing excessive sedation and without causing dependence or tolerance. The sedation induced by phenothiazines differs markedly from that induced by the sedative-hypnotic compounds (see Figure 3.1 in Chapter 3). Even massive doses do not produce anesthesia. The patient who is in a state of drug-induced indifference can easily be aroused with only mild external stimulation. The phenothiazines do not produce euphoria, and the psychological syndrome induced by these drugs is usually not interpreted as being particularly pleasant. The agitation, restlessness, and hyperactivity of the acute schizophrenic attack are frequently dramatically relieved by treatment with chlorpromazine or other phenothiazines. The delusions and hallucinations associated with the acute paranoid attack are particularly sensitive to such treatment. Slightly less susceptible to phenothiazine treatment are the apathy and withdrawal states seen in certain psychotic persons.

The behavioral effects of the phenothiazines may be demonstrated in an animal trained to make a conditioned response. For instance, a rat may be placed in a cage on a wire grid and immediately after a buzzer is sounded, subjected to a small electric shock. The rat will quickly climb a pole to escape the shock. Within very few trials, the animal will learn to associate the buzzer with the electric shock and will climb the pole whenever it hears the buzzer (a *conditioned-avoidance* response). After very small doses of chlorpromazine, the rat will take no notice of the buzzer but will still be able to escape the shock by climbing the pole.

Chlorpromazine is said to block conditioned-avoidance behavior. Other drugs able to block conditioned-avoidance responses are also useful antipsychotic agents, and still others are being tested. Traditional sedative-hypnotic drugs such as the barbiturates, chlordiazepoxide (Librium), or meprobamate (Equanil) do not block conditioned-avoidance responses; instead they depress the response to the buzzer and the response to the shock to approximately the same extent.

The mechanism responsible for this blockage of conditioned avoidance is not entirely understood, but there is evidence that the unresponsiveness to external stimuli (such as the buzzer) is a result of the action of the phenothiazines on the ascending reticular activating system (ARAS) in the brainstem. The ARAS samples all inputs from the senses into the brain. Sensory input activates the ARAS, which in turn alerts the cerebrum to receive information. Whereas the barbiturates and other sedative-hypnotic compounds *directly* depress the neurons in the ARAS, the phenothiazines appear to depress the input into the ARAS. Thus, while the patient is still awake (for it is not the ARAS that is depressed), there is decreased sensory input into the ARAS, so the ARAS does not alert the cerebrum and the cerebrum is unprepared to receive input. The cerebral cortex is then insensible to incoming sensory information.

Side Effects and Toxicity

The phenothiazines differ from the barbiturates not only in their medical uses and behavioral actions but also in their toxicities. In contrast to the barbiturates and other sedative-hypnotics, the phenothiazines are not likely to cause death by respiratory depression. Massive doses may be ingested without producing a significant depression of respiration. The compounds are frequently used in large doses for prolonged periods of time. The side effects associated with the use of these compounds, however, are many, and some invariably accompany the therapeutic use of these drugs.

Phenothiazines produce a variety of disturbances of movement, including tremors, muscle rigidity, walking disorders, and involuntary movements. Other side effects include increased heart rate, dry mouth, blurred vision, and constipation. More serious side effects are altered pigmentation of the skin, pigment deposits on the eye, permanently impaired vision, hormone changes, allergic reactions, and possible liver dysfunction (jaundice). These responses are significant clinical problems, since patients who are not in hospitals tend to refrain from taking their medicine in order to avoid the side effects and inevitably suffer a return of psychotic behavior.

Tolerance and Dependence

One of the positive attributes of the phenothiazines is that they do not appear to be addicting. Tolerance does not develop, nor does physical or psychological dependence. Psychotic patients may take phenothiazines for years without necessarily having to increase their dose because of tolerance, and if a dose is increased, it is usually done in order to obtain better control of the psychotic episodes. Cessation of these drugs is not followed by symptoms of withdrawal, possibly because it may take up to a year for the compounds to be excreted completely. And because phenothiazines do not induce a state of euphoria, there is little psychological dependence or compulsion to misuse them.

HALOPERIDOL

In 1967, haloperidol (see Figure 7.2) was introduced for sale in the United States as the first of a series of compounds referred to as butyrophenone derivatives. Pharmacologically, haloperidol (Haldol) is similar to the phenothiazines. It inhibits motor activity in animals and blocks conditioned-avoidance behavior. In humans, haloperidol produces sedation, indifference to external stimuli, and a reduction in initiative, anxiety, and activity. Haloperidol, however, is metabolized and excreted at a much faster rate than the phenothiazines, and the drug is almost totally excreted within several days after administration is discontinued.

The mechanism of antipsychotic action of this drug is, like that of the phenothiazines, thought to involve a blockage of dopamine receptors. Haloperidol does not exhibit the serious toxicities occasionally seen with the phenothiazines (jaundice, blood abnormalities, and so on), but the involuntary movements are even more pronounced than those induced by chlorpromazine and other phenothiazines. In general, however, haloperidol is an interesting, effective drug for the treatment of psychoses, and it offers an alternative for patients who may be unresponsive to the phenothiazines.

RESERPINE

Both reserpine (Serpasil) and chlorpromazine are effective in the treatment of psychoses, but the side effects associated with reserpine are more pronounced and make the phenothiazines preferable. The most bothersome side effects of reserpine include mental depression, significant depression of blood pressure, and severe diarrhea. Reserpine, however, is of interest since its mechanism of action has been well delineated and the drug is useful for delineating chemical pathways in the brain and mechanisms that may possibly underlie mental disorders.

The antipsychotic effect of reserpine correlates with a drug-induced depletion of norepinephrine (NE) and other amines from the central nervous system. Reserpine blocks the uptake of the NE inside the presynaptic nerve terminal into the storage granules. This means that intraneuronal NE is exposed to the enzyme MAO, by which it is rapidly metabolized. This depletion of NE by reserpine is so effective that severe mental depression may be induced and may result in suicide. Since the phenothiazines do not deplete NE, their sedative and antipsychotic actions are not accompanied by as much mental depression. This NE-depleting action of reserpine does add further weight to the correlation between norepinephrine and the continuum of behavioral states from depression to mania. Reserpine is currently used in the treatment of psychoses only as a substitute for the phenothiazines in those few patients who cannot tolerate any of the phenothiazine derivatives.

LITHIUM

According to the norepinephrine theory of mania and depression (presented in Chapter 5), drugs that increase the action of NE produce degrees of behavioral stimulation directly related to the amount of NE at the synapse. Therefore, drugs such as amphetamine, cocaine, and the antidepressants, which augment the activity of NE neurons, produce a stimulant or antidepressant effect. Conversely, drugs such as reserpine or lithium, which decrease NE levels, either induce a state of behavioral depression or relieve mania. The latter two agents might therefore be thought to be potentially useful in the treatment of mania. Reserpine, however, by depleting the brain of NE induces mental depression, causes an uncomfortable depression of blood pressure, impairs libido, and may cause a rather severe diarrhea. Its clinical utility in the treatment of mania is obviously limited by these rather bothersome side effects.

In contrast to reserpine, lithium is useful in the treatment of mania, especially as a mood-stabilizing drug when used chronically for the prevention of recurrent manic episodes. Lithium is an alkali metal, like sodium and potassium. The compound was employed in the 1920s as a sedative-hypnotic compound, and in 1940 lithium chloride was available as a salt substitute. This latter use produced disastrous consequences, including deaths. In the late 1940s, after an Australian scientist noted that lithium administered to guinea pigs made these animals lethargic, lithium was administered to manic patients, with somewhat spectacular effects. However, it took over 20 years for this agent to become available in the United States and to be accepted by the medical community as an effective treatment for mania.

Unlike the antipsychotic agents discussed above, lithium in therapeutic doses has almost no discernable psychotropic effect in normal persons. It does not induce sedation and exhibits few effects on the brain aside from its specific action on mania. The drug is not a euphoriant. The mechanism through which lithium exerts its anti-mania effect is still a matter of speculation, but current thought holds that it decreases the release of NE from and increases its reuptake into nerve terminals. The net effect of these actions is to decrease the levels of NE at its receptors in the CNS.

Lithium is rapidly absorbed when administered orally. Peak blood levels are reached within one to three hours and correlations exist between the levels of lithium in the blood and therapeutic efficacy. Since lithium closely resembles normal salt (sodium chloride), when salt intake is lowered or when excessive salt is lost (as through sweating), lithium blood levels rise and intoxication may follow. Therefore, in patients on low salt diets or in all patients exposed to warm weather, lithium blood levels must be closely monitored. Toxic reactions consist primarily of fatigue, muscle weakness, slurred speech, and tremor. At high concentrations, more serious toxic effects consisting of muscle rigidity and coma may be observed.

In spite of these side effects, lithium is a rather safe drug which has provided the physician with a compound specifically effective in the prevention of manic episodes, a disorder that prior to lithium was quite resistant to treatment.

NOTES

1. S. H. Snyder, S. P. Banerjee, H. T. Yamamura, and D. Greenberg, "Drugs, Neurotransmitters, and Schizophrenia," *Science* 184 (1974): 1243–53.

2. S. S. Kety, "Recent Genetic and Biochemical Approaches to Schizophrenia," in *Drug Treatment of Mental Disorders,* L. L. Simpson, ed. (New York: Raven Press, 1976), pp. 1–11.

3. H. L. Klawans, C. Goetz, and R. Westheimer, "The Pharmacology of Schizophrenia," in *Clinical Neuropharmacology,* vol. 1, H. L. Klawans, ed. (New York: Raven Press, 1976), pp. 1–26.

Chapter 8

Psychedelic Drugs: Mescaline, LSD, and Other "Mind-Expanding" Agents

Psychedelic drugs are a group of heterogeneous compounds, all with the ability to induce visual, auditory, or other hallucinations and to separate the individual from reality. These agents may induce disturbances in cognition and in perception and, in some instances, may produce behavioral patterns that have been described as being similar to components of psychotic behavior. Because of this wide range of psychological effects, it is difficult to assign a single term that will adequately classify these agents.

The term *hallucinogen* has been widely used, since most of these agents may induce hallucinations, at least if the dose is high enough. Hallucinogen, however, appears to be a somewhat inappropriate term since it does not adequately describe the range of pharmacological actions of such a diverse group of substances. The term

136

psychotomimetic has been assigned to these compounds, in reference to their alleged mimicking of psychoses or inducement of a psychotic state. However, careful analysis of the action of these drugs indicates that their effects are unlike the behavioral patterns observed during psychotic episodes. It appears that the behavioral responses to high doses of amphetamines (Chapter 5) more closely resemble a true psychotic episode.

Because so far we have no completely appropriate term that briefly yet comprehensively characterizes the pharmacology of these drugs, we must rely on a descriptive term such as *phantasticum* (proposed by Lewin in 1924) or *psychedelic* (proposed by Osmond in 1957) to imply that these agents all have the ability to alter sensory perception and thus may be considered to be "mind expanding."

The psychedelic agents have a long and colorful history. Indeed, many are natural in origin, being derived from plants. Today, however, more are synthetically produced in the laboratory (such as LSD and derivatives of tryptamine and amphetamine). Psychedelics have been used for thousands of years. Because of the effects of these naturally occurring drugs on sensory perception, they were frequently ascribed magical, religious, or mystical properties and used as sacraments in religious rites. For many years, the compounds were primarily restricted to local religious rituals and people in the larger world were barely aware of their existence. Of late, however, the psychedelic agents have been "discovered" and advocated by members of modern society as agents that "enhance perception," "expand reality," "promote personal awareness," and "stimulate or induce comprehension of the spiritual or supernatural." An extremely large assortment of written material is currently available describing these more recent aspects of the use of psychedelic drugs. However, even this brief introduction should indicate that the widespread recreational and nonreligious use of psychedelic agents is a fairly new phenomenon, having developed only within the last couple of decades.

CLASSIFICATION

Since the drugs commonly referred to as being phantastica or psychedelics differ widely in chemical structure, they produce a wide range of behavioral alterations. Thus, their classification by chemical structure is difficult. However, since psychoactive drugs are thought to produce behavioral changes as a result of alterations in the synaptic transmission processes, it is possible to classify these compounds by the transmitter upon which the drug is thought to act or that the drug most closely resembles.

As discussed in Appendix II, several chemical substances are commonly thought to serve as synaptic transmitters within the brain. Such substances include acetylcholine (ACh), norepinephrine (NE), dopamine, and 5-hydroxytryptamine (serotonin). Such compounds as physostigmine and diisopropyl fluorophosphate (DFP) increase the amounts of acetylcholine available at its synapses within the brain and induce nightmares, confusion, delirium, agitation, and slowing of intellectual and motor functions. Thus, physostigmine and DFP may be considered as *acetylcholine psychedelics* (see Table 8.1) since they affect ACh transmission. Besides physostigmine and DFP (both of which increase levels of ACh), there are other psychedelic agents that block ACh neurotransmission, thereby decreasing the activity of ACh. Such drugs include atropine and scopolamine.

In Chapter 5, we discussed the action of amphetamine and cocaine on NE neurons in the brain. The behavioral stimulation induced by amphetamine and cocaine appears to be related to the potentiation of NE. At high doses, mania and a paranoid psychosis are induced and accompanied by delusions, hallucinations, and disturbances in sensory perception. Thus, amphetamine and cocaine

Table 8.1. Classification of Psychedelic Drugs

1. Acetylcholine psychedelics
     Physostigmine
     DFP, Sarin, Soman, Malathion, Parathion
     Atropine
     Scopolamine
     Muscarine

2. Norepinephrine psychedelics
     Mescaline
     DOM (STP), MDA, MMDA, TMA
     Myristicin, elemicin

3. Serotonin psychedelics
     Lysergic acid diethylamine (LSD)
     Dimethyltryptamine (DMT)
     Psilocybin, psilocin, bufotenine
     Ololiuqui (morning glory seeds)
     Harmine

4. Psychedelic anesthetics
     Phencyclidine (Sernyl)
     Ketamine (Ketalar)

might well have been discussed as psychedelic agents as well as behavioral stimulants and should be classified, with the wide variety of compounds structurally similar to NE, as *norepinephrine psyche-delics*. As Table 8.1 shows, this classification includes mesca-line, DOM (also called STP), TMA, MDA, MMDA, and certain drugs obtained from nutmeg (myristicin and elemicin). All of these compounds differ from one another and from amphetamine and cocaine in the relative intensity of psychedelic action and behavioral stimulation. Amphetamine and cocaine produce more behavioral stimulation than psychedelic action, whereas the reverse is true for the NE psychedelics listed in the table.

Serotonin, as discussed in Appendix II, appears to be involved in (among other things) sensory perception. The synthesis of lysergic acid diethylamide (LSD) and the discovery of its hallucinogenic prop-erty and its structural resemblance to serotonin initiated a class of psychedelics that is presented in Table 8.1 as *serotonin psychedelics*, a group that includes psilocybin and psilocin (both from the magic mushroom, *Psilocybe mexicana*), dimethyltryptamine (DMT), and bufotenine (isolated from the poisonous mushroom known as fly-agaric, or *Amanita muscaria*).

Finally, there is a fourth classification of psychedelic drugs referred to as the *psychedelic anesthetics*. These agents, phencyc-lidine and ketamine, are structurally unrelated to the other psyche-delic compounds and, to date, the neurotransmitters upon which these compounds exert their activity· have yet to be identified. The structural relations between these three transmitters and the various psychedelic drugs are presented in figures 8.1, 8.2, 8.3, and 8.4.

PSYCHEDELICS ACTING ON ACETYLCHOLINE NEURONS

The activity of acetylcholine (ACh) in the body can be altered through at least three mechanisms. First, ACh levels can be *increased* by drugs that inhibit the enzyme that normally destroys the transmit-ter. Second, ACh activity can be *decreased* by drugs that block the ACh receptors, limiting the access of ACh to its receptors. Third, some drugs will directly stimulate ACh receptors, mimicking the action of the transmitter. Specific drugs that produce these effects are discussed below. (More extensive discussion of ACh neurotransmis-sion may be found in Appendix II.)

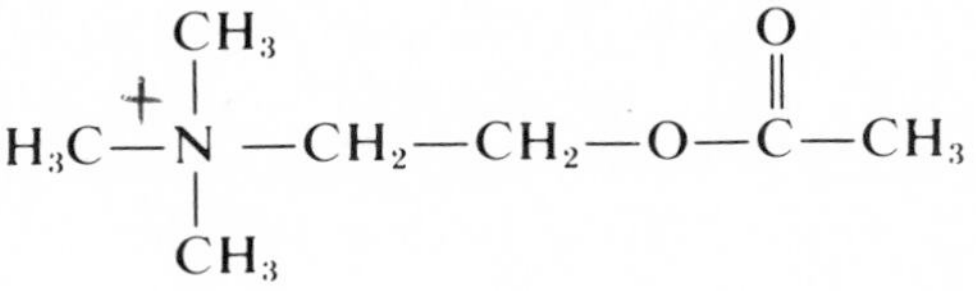

CH₃ structures...

$$\underset{\overset{|}{CH_3}}{\overset{\overset{CH_3}{|}}{H_3C - \overset{+}{N}}} - CH_2 - CH_2 - O - \overset{\overset{O}{\|}}{C} - CH_3 \qquad \text{Acetylcholine}$$

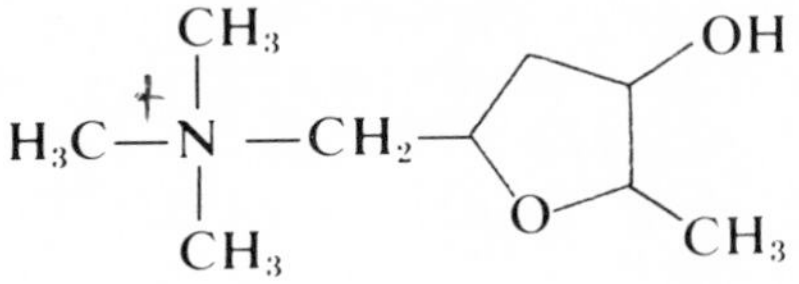

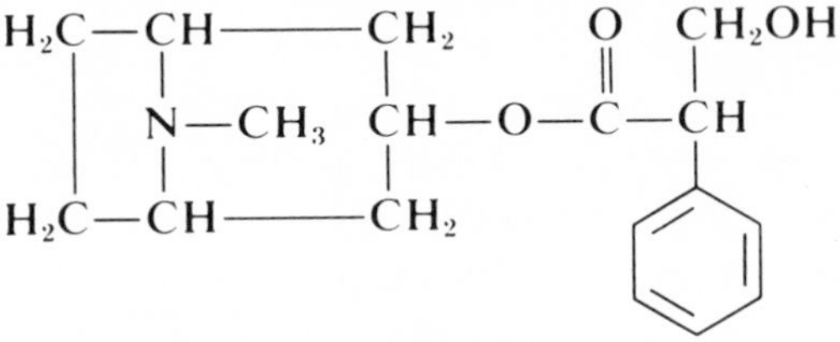

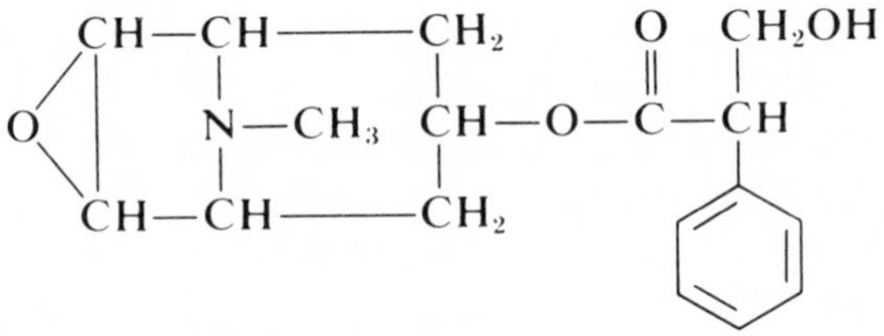

$$\underset{\overset{|}{CH_3}}{\overset{\overset{CH_3}{|}}{H_3C - \overset{+}{N}}} - CH_2 - \text{(tetrahydrofuran ring with OH and CH}_3\text{)} \qquad \text{Muscarine}$$

Atropine (tropane structure):

H₂C—CH——CH₂   O   CH₂OH
        N—CH₃ CH—O—C—CH   Atropine
H₂C—CH——CH₂   (phenyl)

Scopolamine (tropane structure with epoxide):

CH—CH——CH₂   O   CH₂OH
O   N—CH₃ CH—O—C—CH   Scopolamine
CH—CH——CH₂   (phenyl)

Figure 8.1. Structural formulas of acetylcholine (a chemical transmitter), muscarine, atropine, and scopolamine. The latter are three psychedelic drugs thought to act on acetylcholine neurons.

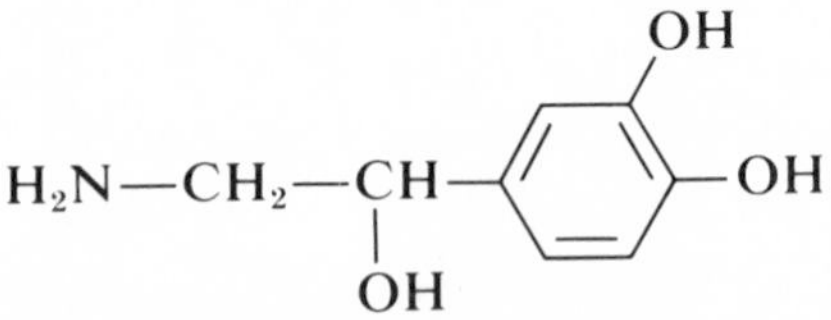

$$H_2N - CH_2 - \underset{\overset{|}{OH}}{CH} - \text{(benzene ring with OH, OH)} \qquad \text{Norepinephrine}$$

Figure 8.2. Structural formulas of norepinephrine (a chemical transmitter) and seven psychedelic drugs. These seven are structurally related to norepinephrine and thought to exert their psychedelic actions through alterations of transmission at norepinephrine synapses in the brain.

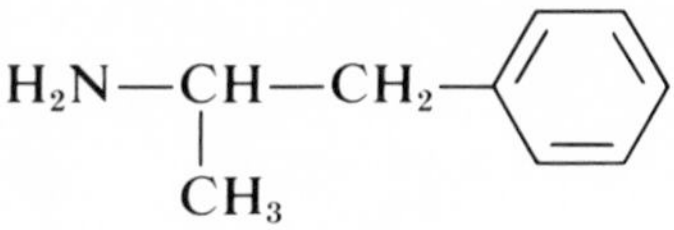

Amphetamine

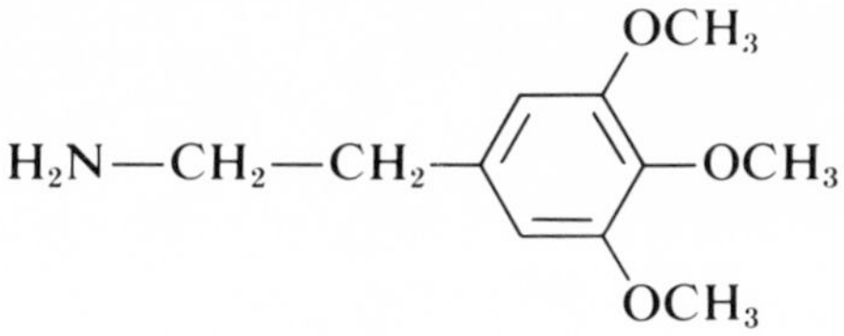

Mescaline

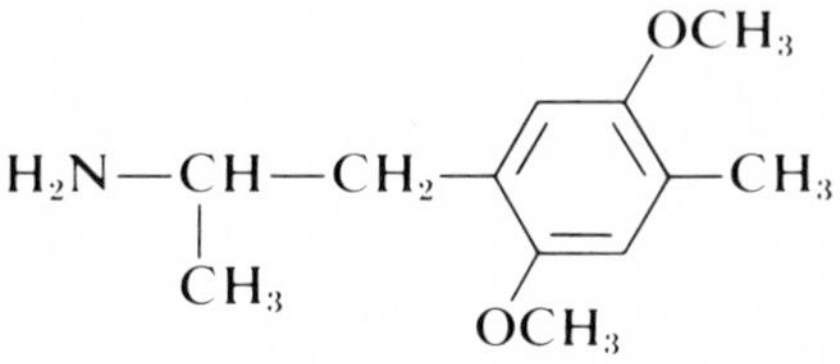

H₂N—CH—CH₂— ... —CH₃   DOM (STP)

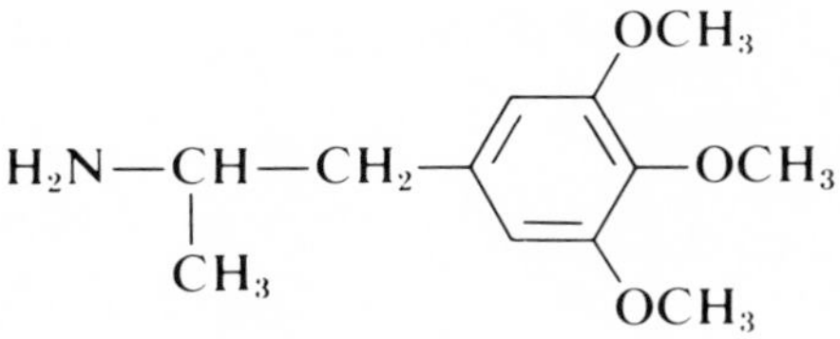

H₂N—CH—CH₂— ... —OCH₃   TMA

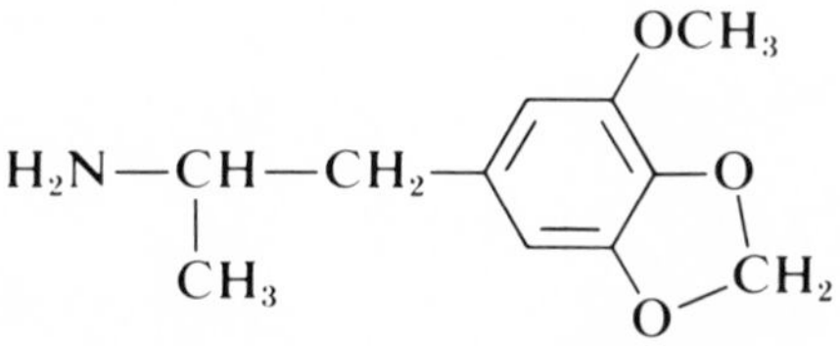

H₂N—CH—CH₂— ... MMDA

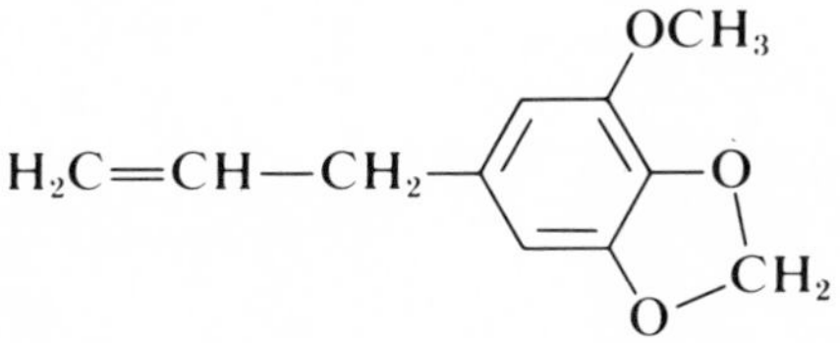

H₂C=CH—CH₂— ... Myristicin

H₂C=CH—CH₂— ... Elemicin

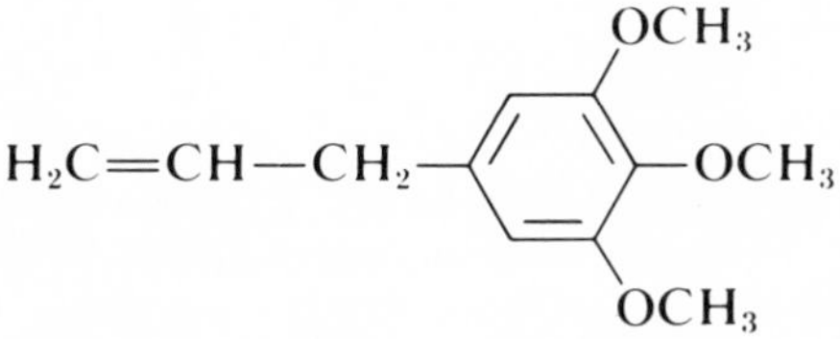

Figure 8.2. (continued)

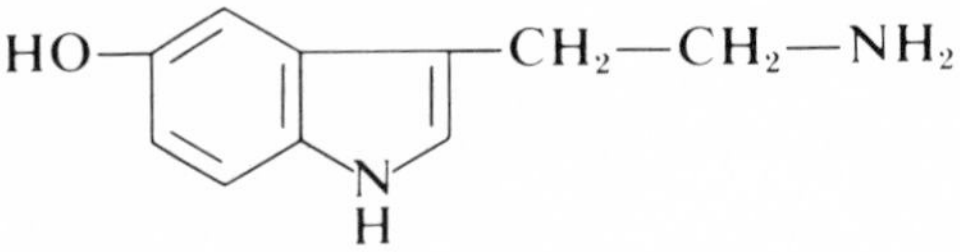

Serotonin

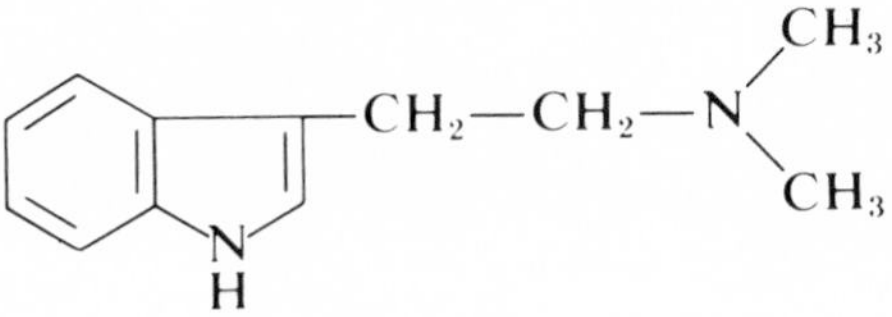

DMT

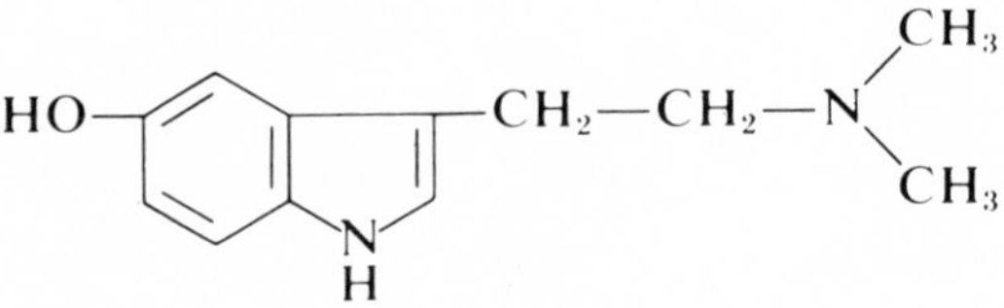

Bufotenine

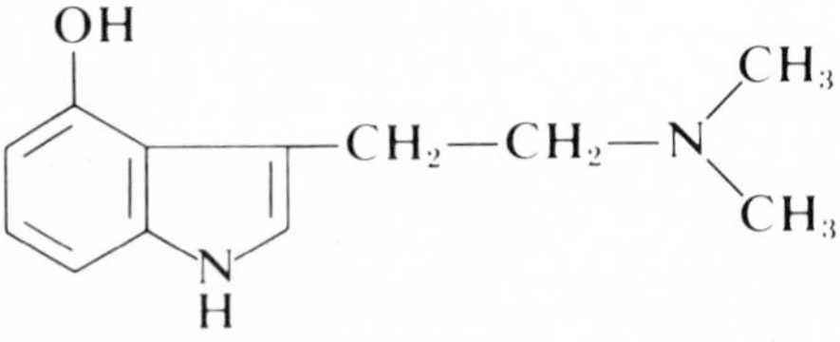

Psilocin

Figure 8.3. Structural formulas of serotonin (a chemical transmitter) and six psychedelic drugs. These six are structurally related to serotonin and thought to exert their psychedelic actions through alterations of serotonin synapses in the brain. Although LSD is structurally much more complex than serotonin, the basic similarity of the two molecules is apparent.

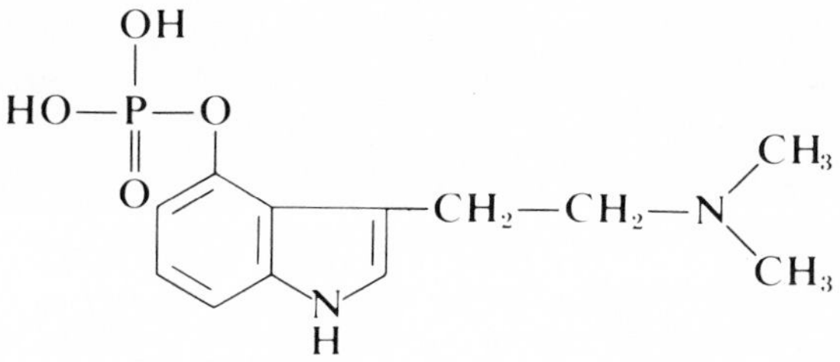

Psilocybin

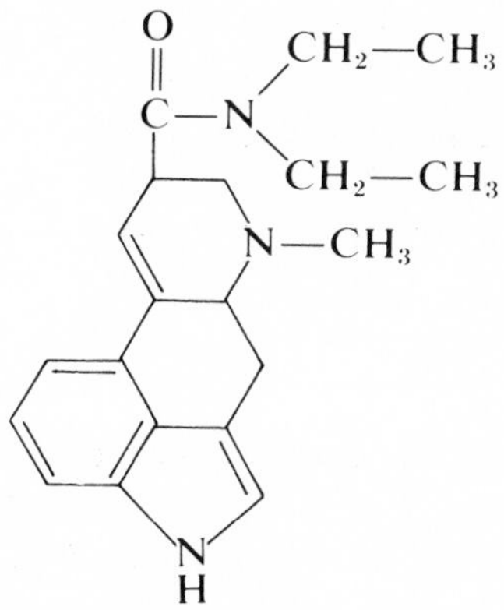

LSD

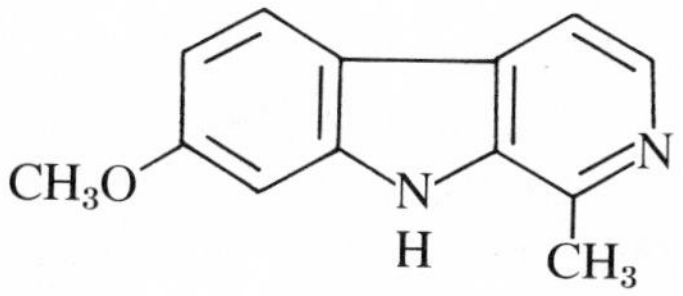

Harmine

Figure 8.3 (continued)

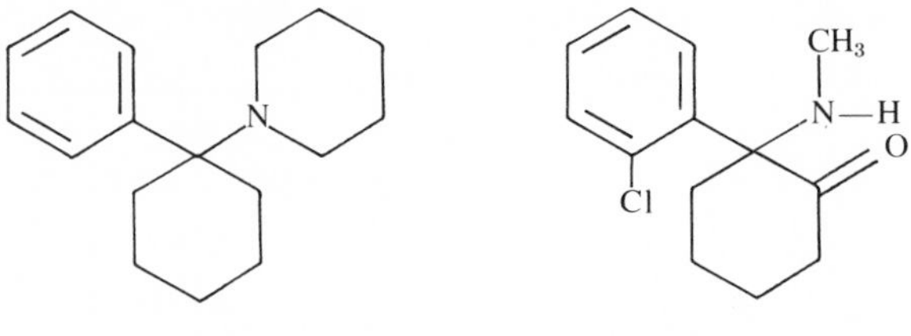

Phencyclidine (Sernyl)   Ketamine (Ketalar)

Figure 8.4. Structural formulas of phencyclidine and ketamine.

Acetylcholinesterase (AChE) Inhibitors

Acetylcholinesterase (AChE) is the enzyme responsible for terminating the transmitter action of ACh both within the brain and in the peripheral nervous system. Drugs that have the ability to inhibit or inactivate AChE are called *anticholinesterases* or *AChE inhibitors*. As a result of AChE inhibition, ACh accumulates in the synaptic cleft and exerts a stronger or more prolonged action. Since these ACh synapses are widely distributed in the brain and peripheral nervous system, it is not surprising that AChE inhibitors produce a wide variety of effects on both the brain and the body.

HISTORICAL BACKGROUND

The prototype AChE inhibitor is a drug called physostigmine, which occurs naturally and was originally obtained from the Calabar bean or ordeal bean *(Physostigma venenosum)* of the Calabar region of Nigeria. This bean was once used by native tribes of West Africa as an ordeal poison. As a test of guilt, a suspect was forced to swallow the beans. If he died, his guilt was proved. If he were confident of his innocence and ate the beans rapidly, he would promptly vomit and survive the ordeal. (It is rumored, however, that proof of innocence or guilt was not always left to chance. Apparently, a placebo was given to those judged to be innocent by the tribal elders in order that justice might not miscarry.)

In the mid-1800s, the Calabar bean was taken to England and studied by several English pharmacologists. Physostigmine was isolated as the active ingredient in the bean and introduced into medicine for the treatment of glaucoma (a disease resulting from increased pressure inside the eye). Subsequently, synthetic AChE inhibitors were produced. It was found that they increased the strength of muscular contraction, so they were used in the treatment of myasthenia gravis (a disease characterized by weakness of the skeletal muscles).

More recently, a new type of AChE inhibitor has been synthesized. The newer agents produce extremely long-lasting inhibition of AChE, to the extent of being irreversible in their action. These substances are compounds such as diisopropyl fluorophosphate (DFP), malathion, parathion, sarin, and soman. Because of their toxicity, some of these irreversible AChE inhibitors are widely used as agricultural insecticides. Because these compounds are toxic not only to insects but also to humans, their use as insecticides has been responsible for an increasing number of accidental poisonings and deaths, especially among field workers. Sarin and soman, among the most potent synthetic toxic and lethal agents known, have been stockpiled for use as nerve gases in chemical warfare.

PHARMACOLOGICAL EFFECTS

The effects of AChE inhibitors in the body are predictable if one knows the location and function of ACh synapses throughout the body. However, since we have very little information about either the location or function of the brain's ACh synapses, we cannot predict the effects of AChE inhibitors on the brain. In the body, AChE inhibitors block ACh synapses and induce any or all of the following effects: constriction of the pupil, constriction of the bronchi, contraction of the bladder and intestinal muscle, profuse salivation and sweating, decreased blood pressure with a slowing of the heart rate, and increased muscle tone followed by paralysis of respiratory muscles, which leads to failure of respiration and eventually death. In the brain, behavioral alterations induced by AChE inhibition consist of anxiety, restlessness, dreaming, nightmares, delirium, and insomnia.

With higher doses, behavioral effects include depression, drowsiness, confusion, uncoordination, ataxia, slurring of speech, convulsions, coma, and paralysis of the medulla, which leads to failure of respiration and death. The respiratory failure that can result in death can therefore be produced by either of two means: by direct paralysis of the respiratory muscles or by paralysis of the respiratory control center in the brainstem.

Since these agents block the enzyme that destroys ACh, ACh accumulates at the synapse. A true antidote would remove the AChE inhibitor from the enzyme AChE, thus restoring the enzyme's ability to metabolize the transmitter. Such antidotes are available for certain AChE inhibitors, although usually available only in hospital emergency rooms. An incomplete antidote might block the action of ACh at the receptor, although it could not regenerate the enzyme. ACh would still be available in excess (owing to AChE inhibition), but it is prevented from reaching its receptor. One such incomplete antidote is atropine, a drug that blocks many of the ACh receptors both in the brain and in the body.

The wide range of behavioral effects of AChE inhibitors (including their ability to induce delirium, nightmares, vivid dreaming, and so on) dictates their inclusion as psychoactive drugs. However, because of their extreme toxicity and numerous side effects, these agents are seldom encountered as drugs of abuse, because the compulsion to misuse them is low and the risks associated with their use outweigh the benefits received.

Blockers of ACh Receptors (Anticholinergic Drugs)

AChE inhibitors exert their effects by increasing ACh activity as a result of increasing the concentration of ACh at the ACh receptors. The drugs to be discussed now (atropine and scopolamine) decrease ACh activity by blocking ACh receptors and consequently preventing transmission across these synapses.

HISTORICAL BACKGROUND

The history of atropine and scopolamine is long and colorful. These two drugs are widely distributed in nature. They are found in especially high concentrations in the plant known as belladonna or deadly nightshade *(Atropa belladonna)*. These drugs are also found in *Datura stramonium* (Jamestown-weed, Jimson-weed, stink-weed, thorn-apple, or devil's-apple), and in *Mandragora officinarum* (mandrake). Scopolamine is found in the shrub *Hyoscyamus niger* (henbane). Preparations of these plants containing atropine and scopolamine have been known and used for centuries. Both professional and amateur poisoners of the Middle Ages frequently used the deadly nightshade as a prime source of poison. In fact, the name *Atropa belladonna* is derived from Atropos, the Greek goddess who supposedly cuts the thread of life. *Belladonna* means "beautiful woman."

If an extract of the plant is applied to the eyelids or, more usually, in the conjunctival sac, the pupils will dilate. To the Romans and Egyptians, dilated pupils were considered beautiful. Even today a woman with dilated pupils is sometimes thought to be more beautiful than a woman with constricted pupils, simply because her eyes look larger. These drugs were often used recreationally for their psychological and behavioral effects. In fact, it is thought that the use of atropine and scopolamine may have persuaded certain individuals that they had the ability to fly, that they were witches.

Plants containing atropine and scopolamine have been used and misused for centuries. Even today, cigarettes made from the leaves of *Datura stramonium* and *Atropa belladonna* are frequently smoked to induce intoxication. Such cigarettes were, until recently, widely sold in drug stores for use in the treatment of asthma, but because they have been misused, they are not now generally available. Throughout the world, leaves of plants containing atropine and scopolamine are still used to prepare intoxicating beverages, and marijuana and opium preparations from the Far East are quite frequently fortified with atropine obtained from *Datura stramonium*.

PHARMACOLOGICAL EFFECTS

In general, the actions of atropine and scopolamine on body function are the opposite of those of the AChE inhibitors. Atropine and scopolamine depress salivation, reduce sweating, dilate the pupils, increase heart rate, and cause loss of tone in the urinary bladder and the gastrointestinal tract. Because these drugs also inhibit the secretion of acid into the stomach, they are frequently used in the medical treatment of ulcers, although their effectiveness is limited by rather significant side effects.

Low doses of scopolamine depress the arousal centers in the ascending reticular activating system (ARAS) of the brain, induce a cortical brain-wave pattern characteristic of sleep, and produce drowsiness, euphoria, amnesia, fatigue, delirium, mental confusion, dreamless sleep, and loss of attention. Low doses of atropine, however, do not seem to affect EEG or behavior. Although atropine and scopolamine can produce delirium and euphoria, because they cloud consciousness, produce amnesia, and do not expand sensory perception, they differ from the norepinephrine and serotonin psychedelics to be discussed later in this chapter.

In brief summary, atropine and scopolamine exert a wide variety of effects, both in the brain and in the body, leading to a sequence of effects ranging from dry mouth, dilated pupils, increased heart rate, and decreased intestinal and bladder tone to behavioral depression, sedation, delirium, mental clouding, and loss of recent memory. Physostigmine will antagonize these effects, but such antagonism is limited by physostigmine's short duration of action.

As psychedelic agents, atropine and scopolamine would seem to be less attractive than those to be discussed later in this chapter because they cloud rather than expand consciousness and impair the memory rather than increase awareness, so that the user cannot remember much of the experience. In addition, the side effects of these compounds tend to limit their recreational use.

Activator of ACh Receptors (Muscarine)

Apart from the Mexican mushroom, *Psilocybe mexicana,* which yields psilocybin and psilocin, there are other mushrooms from which psychoactive drugs may be extracted. One such is fly agaric *(Amanita muscaria),* a mushroom found throughout Europe, especially in Scandinavia (where it is thought to have been used by the Vikings) and northern Siberia. The drug muscarine has been extracted from *Amanita muscaria* along with several other drugs, some of which will be discussed later. The name "fly agaric" is derived, apparently, from the insecticidal properties of the drug. The compound is not lethal to the fly, but apparently when a fly ingests the extract of *Amanita muscaria* it goes into a prolonged stupor and may then be easily killed. Thus, the extract of *Amanita muscaria* (containing muscarine as an active ingredient) is intoxicating and results in a depressed state (a stupor), with concomitant sleep, visions, and delirium. Stupor may be followed by behavioral excitement accompanied by visual and auditory hallucinations and distortions of sensory input. Muscarine is well absorbed orally and appears to be excreted without being metabolized by the liver to an inactive product.

Muscarine itself directly stimulates ACh receptors both in the brain and in the body, inducing profound sweating, greatly increasing salivation, causing pupillary constriction, increasing bladder tone, slowing of heart rate, decreasing blood pressure, and other effects similar to those produced by the AChE inhibitors. This similarity is not unexpected, since both muscarine and the AChE inhibitors increase the activity of ACh neurons.

Mushroom poisoning has been known for centuries. *Amanita muscaria* appears to be responsible for many cases. Symptoms include salivation, sweating, pinpoint pupils, severe abdominal pain, diarrhea, weakness, confusion, and coma. Death may result. Atropine appears to be an effective, though incomplete, antidote.

It should be clear from the description of the effects of *Amanita muscaria* and its active ingredient, muscarine, that this mushroom exerts profound effects on the body in addition to its effect on the brain. These peripheral effects would seem to limit the recreational usefulness of the compound.

PSYCHEDELICS ACTING ON NOREPINEPHRINE NEURONS

In Appendix II, the norepinephrine synapse is discussed as the site of action of several psychoactive drugs and, in chapters 5 and 7, as the site of action of cocaine, amphetamine, the antidepressants, lithium, and possibly even the antipsychotic tranquilizers. We will now discuss the norepinephrine synapses as important sites of action of a large group of psychedelic drugs. As may be seen in Figure 8.2, several psychedelic drugs are structurally similar to both norepinephrine and amphetamine. Such psychedelic agents include mescaline, DOM (also called STP), TMA, MMDA, myristicin, and elemicin. We will discuss each of these agents and pay particular attention to those actions that differentiate these psychedelics from amphetamine and cocaine, which were classified in Chapter 5 as behavioral stimulants rather than as psychedelics.

Mescaline (Peyote)

Peyote *(Lophophora williamsii),* a plant common to the southwestern United States and to Mexico, is a spineless cactus with a small crown or "button" and a long root. For psychedelic use, the crown is ·cut from the cactus and dried to form a hard brown disc, frequently referred to as a mescal button. The dried button may be softened in the mouth and swallowed. Often more than one button may have to be ingested in order to obtain full psychedelic effectiveness.

HISTORICAL BACKGROUND

The use of peyote extends back for centuries—it is known to have been used in the religious rites of the Aztecs. Currently, peyote is the only psychedelic agent that has been sanctioned by the federal government for limited use. It is eaten as an important part of the religious practice of the Native American Church of North America, an organization that claims some one-quarter million members from Indian tribes throughout North America. In order to supply peyote to these Indian tribes, mail-order companies situated in desert regions in the southwestern United States sold the dried buttons at very low prices. In fact, as interest in peyote spread, these mail-order companies occasionally advertised in college newspapers during the late 1950s and early 1960s. In about 1960, interest in peyote became widespread. The interest among college students waned in the mid-

1960s with the rising popularity of a much more powerful psychedelic drug, LSD. However, during the middle to late 1960s, as hostility toward LSD began to develop, hostility toward other psychedelic agents (including peyote) also increased, and laws were passed to control the availability of such drugs.

The Native American Church has so far been able to defeat attempts by the government to outlaw its use of peyote. Members of the church regard peyote as sacramental, much as members of many other churches regard bread and wine as sacramental. It would have to be concluded that the use of peyote for religious purposes is not to be considered "abuse." Indeed, peyote is seldom abused by members of the Native American Church, and the Supreme Court of the United States has ruled that no federal control will interfere with freedom of religion, a ruling that allows the church to continue to use mescaline in religious services.

PHARMACOLOGICAL EFFECTS

The initial research on the active ingredients of the peyote cactus was carried out near the end of the nineteenth century by German pharmacologists. In 1896, mescaline (Figure 8.2) was identified as the active ingredient in peyote. Despite identification of the active ingredient, however, the chemical structure of mescaline was not elucidated until approximately 1918, when its resemblance to norepinephrine was recognized. More recently, because of this structural resemblance, a wide variety of synthetic mescaline and norepinephrine derivatives have been synthesized, and many have psychedelic properties.

Taken orally, mescaline is rapidly and completely absorbed, and significant concentrations within the brain are usually achieved within 30 to 90 minutes. The effects of a single dose of mescaline persist for approximately 12 hours. The drug does not appear to be metabolized before excretion.

Presumably because of its resemblance to norepinephrine, low doses of mescaline produce effects similar to those observed during the fight/flight/fright syndrome: dilatation of the pupils, increased blood pressure and heart rate, an increase in body temperature, EEG and behavioral arousal, and other excitatory symptoms, which are also similar to those produced by amphetamine. However, such actions are not the primary effects sought with mescaline. As one writer puts it:

Interest in mescaline centers on the fact that it causes unusual psychic effects and visual hallucinations. The usual oral dose (5 mg/kg) in the average normal subject causes anxiety, sympathomimetic effects, hyperreflexia of the limbs, static tremors, and vivid hallucinations that are usually visual and consist of brightly colored lights, geometric designs, animals and occasionally people; color and space perception is often concomitantly impaired, but otherwise the sensorium is normal and insight is retained.[1]

Why mescaline induces visual hallucinations but amphetamine seldom does is not known—and is puzzling, since mescaline is structurally so similar to amphetamine. Amphetamine may occasionally produce such hallucinations but only if large doses are taken for long periods of time. Such doses concomitantly induce a state of mania, a reaction that rarely occurs when mescaline is taken in hallucinogenic doses. In contrast to atropine and scopolamine, mescaline produces no delirium, amnesia, or clouding of consciousness. Hallucinations are usually clear and vivid.

Mescaline Derivatives (DOM, TMA, MMDA)

The primary structural differences between amphetamine and mescaline occur on the ring portion of the molecule. Numerous compounds similar to mescaline have been synthesized and several possess the ability to enhance or distort sensory perception. The structures of three of these compounds—DOM, TMA, and MMDA —are illustrated in Figure 8.2. To date, these three have not been extensively studied in experiments on laboratory animals, and most reports of their pharmacologic effects come from users. All three derivatives appear to exert effects similar to those induced by mescaline. Low doses of DOM, TMA, or MMDA produce behavioral excitation, increased motor activity, decreased appetite, increased blood pressure and heart rate, increased body temperature, and so on. At higher doses, visual hallucinations and sensory distortions may be induced that are essentially identical to those produced by mescaline.

TMA is a mescaline derivative differing only by the addition of a $-CH_3$ group on to the basic molecule. MMDA is of the same basic structure, differing only very slightly from TMA. DOM is also closely related to mescaline and is often referred to as STP. (These initials apparently stand for "Serenity, Tranquility, and Peace" or "Super-Terrific Psychedelic.") TMA, DOM, and MMDA appear to differ from mescaline, however, in that all three are considerably more toxic than mescaline as doses are increased. Mescaline itself is usually not considered to be very toxic, even in high doses. However, the behavioral responses to the synthetic mescaline derivatives rapidly progress as the dose is increased from behavioral excitation and sensory hallucinations to gross hyperactivity and hyperexcitability, with accompanying disturbances of body function—effects resembling amphetamine toxicity more closely than the sensory disturbances induced by mescaline. High doses produce tremors that may eventually lead to convulsive movements and prostration, which may be followed by death. Since these synthetic compounds are not commercially available through legitimate sources, there is no standardization of dosage or purity. With mescaline this seems to present little problem because of its wide margin of safety, but with the more toxic synthetic mescaline derivatives, the safety range is less and overdoses may occur much more frequently.

Compounds sold on the street as mescaline are often not mescaline but LSD or one of the synthetic mescaline derivatives. Users must be careful *(caveat emptor)* because higher doses of any of these substitutes can be dangerous. Much work remains to be done to determine the safety, dose ranges, and toxicities of these synthetic derivatives of mescaline.

Myristicin and Elemicin

Myristicin and elemicin are two active ingredients in nutmeg and mace that are responsible for the psychedelic action of these spices. Nutmeg and mace, both readily available in grocery stores, are obtained, respectively, from the dried seed and seed coat of the nutmeg tree *(Myristica fragrans)*. Nutmeg and mace are occasionally encountered as drugs of abuse when no other compounds are available. Ingestion of large amounts (between 1 and 2 teaspoons, usually brewed in a tea) may, after a delay of 2 to 5 hours, induce euphoria and changes in sensory perception, including visual hallucinations.

Considering the close structural resemblance of myristicin and elemicin to mescaline (Figure 8.2), these psychedelic actions are not unexpected. The problem with nutmeg and mace, however, is that these spices induce many unpleasant side effects, including vomiting, nausea, and tremors. Once people have tried nutmeg or mace for its psychedelic action, the side effects usually dissuade them from trying it a second time. The effects of myristicin and elemicin on the brains of experimental animals have not yet been delineated, although the literature indicates that the time course of intoxication is quite long. Further discussion of myristicin intoxication may be found in the symposium edited by Efron.[2]

PSYCHEDELICS ACTING ON SEROTONIN NEURONS

In Appendix II, we discuss the role of serotonin (5-hydroxy-tryptamine, or 5-HT) as a neurotransmitter actively involved in the regulation of body temperature, sleep, and sensory perception. Interest in the actions of serotonin in the brain arose in the late 1950s when it was found that reserpine (see Chapter 7), in addition to decreasing the levels of norepinephrine in the brain, decreased serotonin levels. Theories arose that mental illness (especially schizophrenia) could be caused by abnormalities of transmission between serotonin neurons. These theories were supported by the observation that a number of hallucinogenic compounds were found structurally to resemble serotonin. Figure 8.3 shows that dimethyltryptamine (DMT), bufotenine, psilocin, and psilocybin resemble serotonin in the same way that amphetamine, mescaline, myristicin, and the synthetic mescaline derivatives resemble norepinephrine. Even LSD and harmine are structurally similar to serotonin. (However, the hypothesis that the psychedelic effects induced by this group of agents is due to an action on serotonin neurons has not yet been conclusively proven.) When the serotonin psychedelics are compared with the norepinephrine psychedelics, it appears that the former induce more powerful emotional and sensory experiences but seldom induce the behavioral excitation, mania, and psychosis of amphetamine.

Lysergic Acid Diethylamide (LSD)

In the 1960s and early 1970s, lysergic acid diethylamide (LSD) became one of the most remarkable and controversial drugs known. LSD, in doses that are so small that they might even be considered infinitesimal, is capable of inducing remarkable psychological changes with relatively few alterations in the general physiology of the body. This absence of physiological effects distinguishes LSD from the naturally occurring psychedelics.

HISTORICAL BACKGROUND

LSD was first synthesized in 1938 by Albert Hoffmann, a chemist at the Sandoz Laboratories in Basel, Switzerland. The compound was developed as part of an organized research program seeking to investigate the possible therapeutic uses of a group of compounds obtained from ergot, a natural product derived from a fungus *(Claviceps purpurea)* that grows as a parasite on rye in grainfields of Europe and North America. Epidemics resulting from ingestion of ergot-contaminated grain were reported to consist of bloodless gangrene of the limbs with agonizing burning sensations. In the Middle Ages the disease was called Holy Fire or St. Anthony's Fire, the latter name, according to one account, "being in honor of the saint at whose shrine relief was said to be obtained. The relief that followed migration to the shrine of St. Anthony was probably real, for the sufferers received a diet free of contaminated grain during their sojourn to the shrine."[3] The active products extracted from ergot are derivatives of lysergic acid. The pharmacological actions of these lysergic acid derivates do not usually include hallucinations but do include constriction of blood vessels (which restricts blood flow to the limbs, causing gangrene) and increased contraction of the uterus. Therapeutically, ergot alkaloids are used in the treatment of migraine headache and to control postpartum hemorrhage.

Early pharmacological studies of LSD in animals failed to reveal anything unusual, and the compound was almost forgotten. The psychedelic action was neither sought or expected since most derivatives of ergot are not psychoactive. LSD remained on the laboratory shelf unnoticed from 1938 until 1943, when Dr. Hoffmann had an unusual experience that he later described as follows:

> In the afternoon of 16 April, 1943, . . . I was seized by a peculiar sensation of vertigo and restlessness. Objects, as well as the shape of my associates in the laboratory, appeared to undergo optical changes. I was unable to concentrate on my work. In a dreamlike state I left for home, where an irrestible urge to lie down overcame me. I drew the curtains and immediately fell into a peculiar state similar to drunkenness, characterized by an exaggerated imagination. With my eyes closed, fantastic pictures of extraordinary plasticity and intensive color seemed to surge toward me. After two hours this state gradually wore off.[4]

Hoffmann correctly suspected that his experience must have resulted from accidental ingestion of LSD. He decided to take some of the compound under controlled conditions and describe the experience more completely. Using the dose of other drugs as a guide, he administered what seemed like a minuscule dose (only 0.25 mg, orally). We now know that this dose is many times that required to induce psychedelic effects in most individuals. As a result of his miscalculation, the response was quite spectacular:

> After 40 minutes, I noted the following symptoms in my laboratory journal: slight giddiness, restlessness, difficulty in concentration, visual disturbances, laughing. . . . Later: I lost all count of time. I noticed with dismay that my environment was undergoing progressive changes. My visual field wavered and everything appeared deformed as in a faulty mirror. Space and time became more and more disorganized and I was overcome by a fear that I was going out of my mind. The worst part of it being that I was clearly aware of my condition. My power of observation was unimpaired. . . . Occasionally, I felt as if I were out of my body. I thought I had died. My ego seemed suspended somewhere in space, from where I saw my dead body lying on the sofa. . . . It was particularly striking how acoustic perceptions, such as the noise of water gushing from a tap or the spoken word, were transformed into optical illusions. I then fell asleep and awakened the next morning somewhat tired but otherwise feeling perfectly well.[5]

Four years later, another scientist reported at a meeting in Zurich the results of a clinical investigation of LSD in human subjects. These results essentially confirmed Dr. Hoffmann's original experience. LSD became something of a laboratory and clinical curiosity. In 1949, the first study of LSD in North America in humans was conducted, and, during the 1950s, large quantities of LSD were distributed to pharmacologists and physicians throughout the world for research purposes. A significant impetus to this research was the thought that the effects of LSD might constitute a model psychosis that would provide some insight into the biochemical or physiological processes of mental illness and their treatment.

Subsequently, it was demonstrated that LSD interfered with the transmitter action of serotonin, an observation that led to the hypothesis that serotonin might somehow be involved in mental illness. This hypothesis (although as yet unproven) still seems tenable today. Thus, through the 1950s, LSD was regarded as a tool that might be used to help acquire an understanding of psychoses. LSD has been used as an adjunct to psychotherapy by some therapists to aid patients in verbalizing their problems and in gaining some insight into the underlying causes of the illness, a use that is still much debated.

This early work with LSD on human volunteers was conducted in large medical centers, so the experiments introduced the LSD experience into medical schools and colleges where subjects were paid to participate. LSD propagandists began to appear in the late 1950s and early 1960s, but little attention was paid to them until the activities of Drs. Timothy Leary and Richard Alpert were widely publicized by the mass media. Dr. Leary became the central figure in the national LSD scandal and he instantly became associated with the recreational use of LSD. Indeed, his escapades during the 1960s and 1970s, including his exile in Europe and his subsequent return to the United States in 1973, have continued to add to his notoriety and to inflate the publicity surrounding the use of LSD.

LSD has become one of the most publicized and mysterious drugs of this generation. The drug appeared to reach its peak of popularity in the late 1960s, and today its use appears to have decreased markedly. Considering the long history of other psychedelic agents, it is unlikely that the recreational use of LSD will ever completely disappear. It now seems, however, that the use of LSD in medicine and in psychotherapy will be limited. In the laboratory, LSD will continue to be used to help neuroscientists unravel some of the mysteries of the brain, especially those associated with the role of serotonin as a synaptic transmitter.

ABSORPTION, DISTRIBUTION, METABOLISM, AND EXCRETION

LSD is usually taken orally and is rapidly absorbed. The compound is seldom administered by injection. Since the doses of LSD are so small that several doses could be placed on the head of a pin, the drug is often added to other substances, such as sugar cubes, that may be more easily handled. LSD is rapidly and efficiently distributed throughout the body, easily diffuses into the brain, and readily crosses the placental barrier into the fetus. It appears that the largest amounts of LSD in the body may be found in the liver, where the compound is metabolized before it is excreted. Relatively small levels of the drug are found in the brain, although the compound is so potent that only a few micrograms are needed in order to induce psychedelic effects.

Taken orally, LSD has a rapid onset of action (between 30 and 60 minutes) and its effects persist for approximately 10 or 12 hours.

The mechanism through which LSD exerts its psychedelic action is not known. However, its structural similarity to serotonin and its action on serotonin nuclei within the brain indicate that the drug most likely exerts its effect through actions at serotonin synapses. LSD has been demonstrated to increase the sensitivity of the arousal center in the reticular formation (the ARAS) to incoming sensory information. Unlike amphetamine, LSD does not stimulate this structure directly but somehow alters its receptivity to incoming information such that this information seems to be augmented and expanded, which would account for the apparent expansion of sensory input (especially visual and auditory) experienced during LSD intoxication. Chlorpromazine, because it decreases input into the ARAS, is sometimes used to ameliorate an unwanted or disturbing LSD experience (a "bum trip"). Therapy with chlorpromazine is frequently successful but is certainly not specific, universally predictable, or a panacea for bad trips. Occasionally, chlorpromazine actually intensifies a bad LSD experience. Also, chlorpromazine treatment might fail if the LSD that produced the bad experience were adulterated with other drugs—or were not LSD at all, but a concoction of assorted drugs that might produce bizarre effects.

PHARMACOLOGICAL EFFECTS

Although the LSD experience is characterized primarily by psychological alterations (see below), there are subtle physiological changes that bear discussion. LSD causes a slight increase in body temperature, dilates the pupils, slightly increases heart rate and blood pressure, produces sweating and chills, increases levels of glucose (sugar) in the blood, occasionally produces "goose pimples," headache, nausea, vomiting, and other effects that, although noticeable, seldom interfere with the psychedelic experience and are seldom serious.

LSD is known to possess a low level of toxicity. Deaths due to overdose have not been reported. Similarly, it has not been demonstrated that permanent brain damage may be induced, even by repeated administration of high doses of LSD. It would seem that the drug is nonlethal, in spite of the profound psychological alterations that may be induced by minuscule doses. This is not to say, however, that LSD is innocuous and should be freely available. While the drug may be comparatively safe, both short- and long-term alterations in the psyche of the user and possible adverse effects on the fetus must be considered. The social complications arising from possible widespread and indiscriminate LSD use should also be considered.

PSYCHOLOGICAL EFFECTS

While the physiological alterations produced by LSD are usually quite minor and predictable, the psychological effects are not as predictable. They may be influenced by a variety of factors, including the personality of the users, their expectations of what the drug will produce, their previous use of LSD and psychoactive drugs, their attitudes toward use of LSD or any other illicit drug, their motivations for using the drug, the setting in which the drug is administered, and the individuals with whom they will interact during the LSD experience. The psychological effects induced by LSD are not necessarily directly related to the dose that is administered, since many of the psychological alterations induced are relatively unaffected by increases or decreases in dosage.

Because of these variables, it is difficult to predict the exact psychological experience that will be felt by an individual user on a given occasion. Thus, it is quite difficult to list in order the intensity of responses that might communicate to the reader the essentials of the experience. LSD experiences have been described in innumerable lay publications with glowing eloquence by authors with most imaginative and inventive minds. The essentials of an LSD experience, however, include significant alterations in mood and emotion in which laughter or sorrow may easily be evoked, even simultaneously. Both euphoria and dysphoria can be experienced, even by the same individual during the same trip. The principal psychological effects involve perceptual changes, especially visual hallucinations and distortions. Perceptual changes, according to Jarvik,

> . . . are usually visual and tactile in nature and may consist in either distortions or hallucinations. Auditory manifestations are rather rare. This is in contrast to the high incidence of auditory hallucinations in the naturally occurring psychosis. Intellectual processes are also impaired by the drug, resulting in confusion and difficulty in thinking. The intellectual impairment may be primary but may also result from emotional and motivational changes produced by the compound.[6]

Objects that are visualized may be seen in strange, distorted ways, with clear-cut shapes and brilliant colors. The descriptions of the original LSD trip experienced by Hoffmann (discussed earlier) are probably the most lucid and exciting yet presented, possibly because the chemist had no preconceived notions about what to expect.

TOLERANCE AND DEPENDENCE

Tolerance (a need to increase the dose in order to obtain the same effect) of both the psychological and physiological alterations induced by LSD readily develops. *Cross tolerance* between LSD and other psychedelic agents, such as mescaline and psilocybin, may also develop. An individual who has developed tolerance to LSD will usually show a diminished response to mescaline or psilocybin. Cross tolerance between LSD and marijuana has not been demonstrated.

It has become quite clear that *physical dependence* on LSD does not develop, even when the drug is used repeatedly over a prolonged period of time. In fact, most heavy users of the drug say that they ceased using LSD because they tired of it, had no further need for it, or had had enough. Even when the drug is discontinued because of concern about bad trips, or about physical or mental harm, withdrawal signs are not exhibited.

It appears that *psychological dependence* may occur in those few individuals who have become preoccupied with the drug. Normally, however, such preoccupation seems to run its course and is self-limiting. Most users eventually cease using LSD and return to other less potent psychedelic agents or to the more traditional sedative-hypnotic compounds such as alcohol or marijuana.

ADVERSE REACTIONS AND TOXICITY

The adverse reactions and toxicities attributed to LSD generally fall into four categories: (1) the effects on the psychological state of the user, (2) the possibility of permanent damage to the brain, (3) the possible effects on the fetus when the drug is taken by a pregnant woman, and (4) the deleterious effects upon society in general as a result of widespread use.

At present, scientific information is limited, but much emotion has been generated for and against the existence of such toxicities. For example, there is considerable evidence (some valid and much invalid) to indicate that *extremely high* doses of LSD may cause chromosome breakage. However, similar chromosome breakage may be induced by caffeine, aspirin, many other drugs, X-rays, fever, and viral infections. Even if LSD *in normal doses* should increase the rate of chromosome breakage, the user or any offspring will not necessarily be affected. In fact, clinical data indicate that the incidence of fetal abnormalities occurring in offspring of LSD users does not differ from the incidence in the normal population. While there is *some* evidence of increased incidence of structural abnormalities in infants born of parents who use LSD, the variety of other drugs also used by these same parents precludes assignment of cause to any specific compound. The state of nutrition and lack of prenatal care must also be considered in such populations of users.

Psychoactive drugs (including LSD) *do* cross the placental barrier and have free access to the developing fetus. One should be aware that LSD or any other psychoactive agent may have some as yet undetermined effect on offspring. While current data indicate that the risk is small, the possibility has not been excluded.

Whether long-term, frequent, high-dose use of LSD results in discernible damage to the brain or to any other area of the body has not been determined, although it is generally agreed that experimental use of LSD on only a few occasions does not induce physical damage to either the body or the brain.

It has been demonstrated that when normal individuals are given a battery of psychological tests, then given LSD and re-examined six months later, there does not appear to be residual psychological damage resulting from the drug experience. In fact, these individuals tend to show increases in esthetic appreciation. In an individual who is moderately unstable to begin with, the LSD experience may precipitate psychotic episodes that the user might normally have been able to suppress. Such psychotic episodes may require long-term therapy for the underlying mental disease.

In addition, there is the persistent problem of flashbacks, which may recur weeks or even months after the use of LSD. It is not known how these flashbacks occur or whether LSD induces persistent biochemical alterations that may be responsible for them. The flashback occurs only in a drug-free individual, regardless of how many doses have been used previously. No one has yet been able to produce a flashback in a laboratory animal, and therefore it has not been possible to study flashbacks under controlled laboratory conditions. One may only advise caution and indicate that LSD may produce long-term psychological effects in certain individuals.

Fears of long-term damage to *society* inflicted by widespread use of LSD appear to be unjustified at this time. Within the last few years, the use of LSD has markedly declined, presumably because many who used the drug no longer do so and possibly because the news media no longer find LSD users newsworthy.

There is ample evidence to indicate that LSD induces tolerance to its several effects, but it does not create physical dependence.

Psychological dependence may occur to some extent, since the psychological alterations induced by LSD may lead to a compulsion to reuse the drug. Most users, however, eventually cease taking the drug and return to less potent agents, which would indicate that the compulsion decreases with increased exposure to LSD experiences. Thus, despite the extreme potency and the unusual psychedelic effects that LSD induces, the social use of other psychoactive drugs, such as alcohol, nicotine, amphetamine, barbiturates, tranquilizers, caffeine, and the opiates, should cause more concern.

Dimethyltryptamine (DMT)

Earlier in this chapter, when we discussed the norepinephrine psychedelics (mescaline, DOM, TMA, MMDA, myristicin, and elemicin), their close structural similarity to norepinephrine was stressed. LSD closely resembles serotonin, and the psychedelic effects of LSD are thought to result from alterations in the activity of serotonin neurons. There are various other naturally occurring psychedelic compounds that also closely resemble serotonin and are capable of producing LSD-like effects on the user. One such agent is dimethyltryptamine, DMT (Figure 8.3).

DMT is not extensively used in the United States, but it is widely used in other parts of the world. It is an active principle of various South American snuffs, such as cohoba (prepared from the beans of the *Piptadenia peregrina*) and yopo (a similar product from the West Indies). DMT is partly responsible for the hallucinations and confusional syndrome that follow inhalation of these powders, but the drug bufotenine, which is also present (to be discussed shortly), contributes to the effect. Unlike LSD, DMT is not absorbed into the bloodstream when taken orally and therefore is usually inhaled through the lungs either as a powder or as a smoke.

The psychedelic properties of DMT appear to result predominantly from alterations in visual perception or the occurrence of true hallucinations. Euphoria and behavioral excitability often accompany the sensory alterations. The duration of action of DMT is extremely short, usually only about an hour or two, hence its slang name, "businessmen's LSD."

At the moment, little information is available about the development of tolerance to or dependence upon DMT, but it is expected that it would differ little from LSD. Similarly, it could be predicted that cross-tolerance would occur between LSD and DMT, but this has not been investigated.

Psilocybin and Psilocin

The structures of psilocybin and psilocin were presented in Figure 8.3. The reader might note their close similarity to each other, to DMT and LSD, and to serotonin. Psilocybin and psilocin are the psychedelic agents obtained from the Mexican magic mushroom *(Psilocybe mexicana,* also referred to as Teonanacatl or God's Flesh). These Mexican mushrooms have a long and colorful history of religious and sacramental use throughout Central America.

Psilocin and psilocybin are the active drugs in the mushroom, and they are approximately 1 percent as potent as LSD—that is, 10 mg of psilocybin would produce the same degree of pharmacological action as 0.1 mg (100 μg) of LSD. Unlike DMT, psilocin and psilocybin *are* effectively absorbed when taken orally, and the mushrooms are eaten raw in order to induce psychedelic effects. Even today, these mushrooms continue to be used throughout Central America, although their popularity has not spread to the United States.

For a long while it was thought that psilocin and psilocybin were both pharmacologically active. However, as can be seen from Figure 8.3, the two compounds differ only in that psilocybin contains a molecule of phosphoric acid. What appears to happen after the mushroom has been ingested is that the phosphoric acid is removed from psilocybin, producing psilocin, the active psychedelic agent.

Although the psychedelic effects of *Psilocybe mexicana* have long been part of Indian folklore, the first detailed description of *Psilocybe* intoxication was not obtained until 1955, when Gordon Wasson, a New York banker, traveled through Mexico, mingled with native tribes, and was allowed to participate in a *Psilocybe* ceremony and eat the magic mushroom. Of the mushroom, Wasson said:

> It permits you to travel backwards and forward in time, to enter other planes of existence, even to know God. . . . Your body lies in the darkness, heavy as lead, but your spirit seems to soar and leave the hut, and with the speed of thought to travel where it listeth, in time and space, accompanied by the shaman's singing . . . at least you know what the ineffable is, and what ecstasy means. Ecstasy! The mind harks back to the origin of that word. For the Greeks, *ekstasis* meant the flight of the soul from the body. Can you find a better word to describe this state?[7]

The hallucinations and distortions of time and space are similar to those produced by LSD. The duration of action of *Psilocybe,* however, is much shorter (between 2 and 4 hours) than the duration of action of LSD. Cross tolerance occurs between psilocybin, LSD, and also mescaline. Like LSD, side effects always precede development of the psychedelic action. Users feel symptoms associated with the fight/flight/fright response concomitantly with the psychological effects so vividly described by Wasson.

Psilocybin is not as potent as LSD, and it is somewhat easier to adjust the dose to reach a desired level of drug effect. Low doses of psilocybin (up to 4 or 5 mg) induce a pleasant experience with mental relaxation. Higher doses (to 15 mg) induce perceptual alterations, with occasional hallucinations.

Bufotenine

Earlier in this chapter, we discussed *Amanita muscaria* and one of its psychoactive drugs, muscarine. *Bufotenine* is another drug that is found in *Amanita,* although the amounts are small. More significant amounts of bufotenine may be obtained from the secretion of the skin and parotid glands of toads. Bufotenine may also be found (as is DMT) in the seeds of the tree *Piptadenia peregrina,* which grows in Haiti and Venezuela. These seeds are pulverized and inhaled as snuff. Such preparations are referred to by various names, including yopo, parica, epena, and cohoba.

From Figure 8.3, one may note the close similarity of bufotenine to psilocin, DMT, psilocybin, LSD, and serotonin. Thus, it is not unexpected that the symptoms of intoxication following inhalation of a smoke or powder containing bufotenine are similar to the effects produced by other serotonin psychedelics. The fight/flight/fright responses are induced, followed by a period of excitation, followed finally by a state of stupor and sleep. Pharmacologically, bufotenine (in doses of 1 to 16 mg) may induce visual distortions together with a feeling of relaxation and light-weightedness. Hallucinations may or may not occur.

The side effects of bufotenine (increased blood pressure and heart rate, blurred vision, increased muscle tone, and so on) are greater than those produced by psilocybin or DMT and are often quite bothersome. Thus, bufotenine is more toxic than psilocybin and induces deficits of motor function with ataxia (staggering), minor paralysis, and muscular rigidity. Since these side effects may be frightening to the user, the drug is remarkably uncomfortable to take and such effects might be confused with hallucinations.

Ololiuqui (Morning Glory)

Ololiuqui is yet another naturally occurring agent used by Central American and South American Indians, both as an intoxicant and as a hallucinogen. The drug is used ritually as a means of communicating with the supernatural, as are extracts of most plants that contain drugs of psychedelic potency. Use of ololiuqui seeds in Central and South America was first described by the Spaniard Hernandez who stated that "when the priests wanted to commune with their Gods . . . [they ate ololiuqui seeds and] a thousand visions and satanic hallucinations appeared to them."[8]

The seeds were analyzed in Europe by Albert Hoffmann and several ingredients were identified. One ingredient was lysergic acid amide (*not* lysergic acid diethylamide, LSD). The lysergic acid amide that Hoffmann identified is approximately one-tenth as active as LSD as a psychoactive agent. However, considering the extreme potency of LSD, lysergic acid amide is still quite potent.

Accompanying the psychedelic action of ololiuqui are the usual side effects of the serotonin psychedelics: nausea, vomiting, headache, increased blood pressure, dilated pupils, sleepiness, and so on. These, however, are not usually as intense as those induced by bufotenine.

Harmine

Harmine is a psychedelic agent obtained from the seeds of *Peganum harmala,* a plant native to the Middle East. These seeds have been used for centuries. Intoxication is usually accompanied by nausea and vomiting, sedation and, finally, sleep, and psychic excitement consisting of visual distortions similar to those induced by LSD. Harmine has been relatively well studied in animals, and the reader is referred to Longo's discussion of the drug.[9]

PSYCHEDELIC ANESTHETICS

In Chapter 3, when we discussed the sedative-hypnotic compounds, we stated that all of them were capable of inducing a state of behavioral disinhibition but, because such disinhibition is not usually considered to be hallucinogenic or psychedelic, the sedative-hypnotics are not usually considered to be psychedelic compounds. Within the last decade, however, a new class of anesthetic agents has been introduced. These differ markedly from the traditional sedative-hypnotic agents and appear to resemble more closely the psychedelic compounds. Among such agents are phencyclidine (PCP, Sernyl) and ketamine (Ketalar).

Phencyclidine was synthesized in 1956 and was recommended for clinical trials as an anesthetic in humans in 1957. Earlier investigations of its effects in animals revealed a potent analgesic (pain-relieving) activity and its potential use as a nonbarbiturate, nonnarcotic, intravenous anesthetic agent. However, reports obtained from patients after surgery noted a number of quite severe reactions upon waking from anesthesia. These reactions included agitation, excitement, disorientation, and "hallucinatory" phenomena. In 1965, further human clinical investigation of phencyclidine was discontinued and the compound was marketed commercially as a veterinary anesthetic, primarily for use in primates. The structurally related anesthetic, ketamine (see Figure 8.4), was subsequently developed. Ketamine induced a similar state of anesthesia, but the psychedelic reactions were much less severe. Ketamine was therefore marketed as an anesthetic agent for human use.

In 1967, small amounts of phencyclidine became available through the drug culture, and the drug was referred to in that year as the "PeaCe Pill" (PCP). There was then a sharp decline in phencyclidine use between the years 1971 and 1975, and most PCP during this period was available as a component of various illicit drug mixtures. In 1975, however, there was a resurgence in illicit phencyclidine use. In Detroit, for instance, phencyclidine was reported to be the most commonly found drug when emergency-room records were screened for drug overdoses.

Phencyclidine has appeared on the illicit market in powder, tablet, leaf mixture, and 1 gram "rock" crystal forms. Phencyclidine found on parsley, mint, or other leaves is usually in the form of a "joint." Phencyclidine is commonly sold as "crystal," "angel dust," "PCP," "THC," "cannabinol," or "horse tranquilizer." The most persistent misrepresentation is "THC." When sold as "crystal" or "angel dust" (terms also used for methamphetamine), the drug is usually available in concentrations varying between 50 and 100 percent. When purchased under other names or in concoctions, the amount of phencyclidine drops to a range of 10 to 30 percent. Phencyclidine is usually taken orally, by smoking, snorting, or by intravenous injection. Powdered forms are generally sprinkled on "joints" or sometimes snorted.

The pharmacology of phencyclidine is complicated. This compound (and its close relative, ketamine) does not induce anesthesia in a manner similar to that induced by the sedative-hypnotic drugs discussed in Chapter 3. Phencyclidine and ketamine are frequently referred to as "dissociative anesthetics," since patients may feel dissociated from themselves and from their environment. In humans, phencyclidine appears to be unique among all anesthetics studied. This drug induces an unresponsive state with complete anesthesia, although the eyes remain open (blank stare) and the patient appears to be awake. Significant depression of either respiration or blood pressure is not produced by either phencyclidine or ketamine in anesthetic doses. Toxic doses of these agents may produce severe agitation, muscle rigidity, and generalized seizure activity. Used illicitly, low dose of phencyclidine produce a state of mild agitation or excitement in a patient who appears grossly "drunk" and has a blank stare. The patient may be rigid and unable to speak. In most cases, however, the patient is communicative, although he or she does not respond to pain (these drugs are potent analgesics). In higher doses, a state of coma or stupor in which the eyes remain open is induced. Blood pressure may be elevated and respiration is not depressed. The patient may recover from this state within 1 to 4 hours, although a confusional state may last for 8 to 72 hours.

Massive oral "overdoses," involving up to 1 gram of street-purchased material, have been reported to result in prolonged periods of stupor or coma. This state may last for several days and may be marked by potentially lethal depression of respiration, intense seizure activity, and increased blood pressure. Following this period of stupor, a prolonged recovery phase marked by confusional delusion may last for up to two weeks. In a few cases, this confusional state may be followed by a psychosis lasting several weeks to a few months.

Chronic users of phencyclidine frequently present themselves in hospital emergency rooms with psychiatric problems such as paranoid psychosis, severe depression, anxiety, or concern about brain damage. Indeed, in Washington, D.C., phencyclidine psychosis is presently the leading cause of psychiatric admissions. Whether this drug indeed causes these problems or whether the personality type attracted to high dose or prolonged phencyclidine abuse has one of these underlying problems is as yet unclear.

A number of deaths attributed to phencyclidine overdosage have now been reported. Fourteen deaths associated with phencyclidine have been documented within the period of 1970 to 1975. The cause of death is not clear, although respiratory depression, gen-

eralized seizure activity, and pulmonary edema have all been implicated. For additional readings on phencyclidine, a recent volume is
recommended.[10]

Note from Figure 8.4 that phencyclidine and ketamine are
structurally dissimilar from acetylcholine, norepinephrine, and serotonin. These psychedelic anesthetics cannot therefore be classified as
acting upon any known transmitter chemical in the brain. This unique
situation is not only interesting but offers a pharmacological tool with
which one may study the mechanisms of mental illness. While the
personality changes associated with LSD use are somewhat similar to
those induced by phencyclidine, many of the other features of phencyclidine psychosis are not common to other psychedelic drugs. In
addition, there are reports that phencyclidine may both activate and
mimic schizophrenic psychoses. Some individuals have developed
classic schizophrenia following phencyclidine psychoses. These
observations suggest a relationship between the pharmacology of
phencyclidine and the biochemistry of schizophrenia. Additional research into phencyclidine psychosis may, therefore, further our
understanding of the pathology of schizophrenia and other mental
disorders.

NOTES

1. M. E. Jarvik, "Drugs Used in the Treatment of Psychiatric Disorders,"
   in *The Pharmacological Basis of Therapeutics,* 4th ed., L. S. Goodman
   and A. Gilman, eds. (New York: Macmillan, 1970), p. 195.

2. D. H. Efron, ed., *Ethnopharmacologic Search for Psychoactive Drugs,*
   Public Health Service Publication no. 1645 (Washington, D.C.: U.S.
   Government Printing Office, 1967).

3. P. Brazeau, "Oxytocics," in *The Pharmacological Basis of Therapeutics,* L. S. Goodman and A. Gilman, eds. (New York: Macmillan,
   1975), p. 872.

4. *Interim Drug Report of the Commission of Inquiry into the Nonmedical
   Use of Drugs,* Gerald LeDain, chairman (Ottawa: Information Canada,
   1970), p. 58.

5. *Ibid.,* pp. 58–59.

6. Jarvik, "Drugs Used in the Treatment of Psychiatric Disorders," p. 196.

7. M. E. Crahan, "God's Flesh and Other Pre-Columbian Phantastica,"
   Bulletin of the Los Angeles County Medical Association 99 (1969): 17.

8. Quoted in E. M. Brecher and *Consumer Reports* editors, *Licit and Illicit Drugs* (Mt. Vernon, N.Y.: Consumers Union, 1972), p. 345.

9. V. C. Longo, *Neuropharmacology and Behavior* (San Francisco: W. H.
   Freeman, 1972), pp. 136–41.

10. *Clinical Toxicology,* vol. 9, no. 4 (New York: Marcel Dekker, 1976).

Chapter 9

Marijuana and Hashish: The Ancient Drug of *Cannabis*

Marijuana is an ancient drug. The hemp plant *Cannabis sativa* grows throughout the world and flourishes in most of the temperate and tropical areas. One of humanity's oldest cultivated nonfood plants, it appears to have originated in Asia. The earliest written reference to *Cannabis sativa* dates from approximately 2700 B.C. The substance called *marijuana* is a mixture of the crushed leaves, flowers, and even small branches of both the male and female plants of the species. Hashish is an extract of the plant material.

In both marijuana and hashish, Δ^9-tetrahydrocannabinol (hereafter referred to as THC) is the primary psychoactive agent, although other cannabinols present in much smaller quantities may exert some effect. Since hashish is the extract of the plant, it usually has a higher concentration of THC than does marijuana—anywhere

168

from two to ten times as much. Note that the active ingredient is the same in both preparations; only the amount differs.

In popular literature within the last decade, there has been an explosion of emotional arguments claiming that *Cannabis* is either harmless or else a great danger to the user and to society. Attempting to answer public concern about marijuana, several well-documented reports prepared by various governments have recently become available. The reports have consisted of analyses of the available knowledge about the pharmacological and sociological effects of marijuana and hashish, and the conclusions have tended to be similar despite the polarity and emotion that have been so widely generated within society.

The first major government report was published in 1967. Entitled *Task Force Report: Narcotics and Drug Abuse,* it was prepared by the President's Commission on Law Enforcement and Administration of Justice. This was followed in 1968 by *Cannabis: Report of the British Advisory Committee on Drug Dependence.* In 1970, the Canadian government published the *Interim Report of the Commission of Inquiry into the Non-medical Use of Drugs.* In 1972, two exhaustive reports on marijuana appeared. The Canadian government published a final report, *Cannabis: A Report of the Commission of Inquiry into the Non-medical Use of Drugs,* and the American National Commission on Marihuana and Drug Abuse published *Marihuana: A Signal of Misunderstanding.* The U.S. Department of Health, Education, and Welfare has submitted four annual reports to the Congress on the effects of marijuana on health. Finally, the National Institute on Drug Abuse has sponsored a symposium on the pharmacology of marijuana, and the results of this symposium were recently published in two volumes. References to all these works may be found in the bibliography. These volumes are (at the time of this writing) the latest in a series of objective descriptions of *Cannabis* and its effects.

It is quite likely these reports will not be the last, as public concern about marijuana often tends to run counter to scientific data and conclusions. However, if one examined the historical development of concepts about *Cannabis,* one would see that the recommendations of the Canadian, British, and American governments that the severe penalties for possession of marijuana be relaxed are not new. In fact, in 1894, a 3281-page, seven-volume report entitled *The Indian Hemp Drugs Commission Report* arrived at nearly the same conclusions as those presented some 75 years later. Similarly, Mayor

La Guardia's 1944 report, *The Marihuana Problem in the City of New York* (also called the *La Guardia Committee Report*), reiterated the conclusions of the 1894 report and differs little from the reports presented in 1972. Thus, objective analyses of the effects of *Cannabis* have been with us for some 75 years. However, the public emotion that surrounds marijuana and other *Cannabis* products has tended to cloud objectivity.

CLASSIFICATION

Tetrahydrocannabinol (THC) is a difficult compound to classify. At low to moderate doses, THC is a mild sedative-hypnotic agent resembling alcohol and the antianxiety agents (chlordiazepoxide, diazepam, and meprobamate) in its pharmacological effects. Unlike the sedative-hypnotics, however, higher doses of THC may (in addition to sedation) produce effects similar to a mild LSD experience. Also unlike the sedatives, high doses of THC do not produce anesthesia, coma, or death. Similarly, there appears to be little cross tolerance between THC and LSD on one hand or between THC and the sedative-hypnotic compounds on the other. Thus, the THC contained in the various preparations of *Cannabis* is the only superficially related to either the sedatives or the psychedelics.

Legally, products from *Cannabis sativa* have frequently been classified with the opiates as narcotics. As is well known and appreciated today, marijuana and hashish are *not* narcotics and are pharmacologically quite distinct from the opiates (Chapter 6). *Cannabis* products are currently used in the United States chiefly in the form of marijuana, of which approximately 1 to 3 percent consists of THC. Because marijuana has so little THC, the product at normally encountered doses (one or two cigarettes, or "joints") quite closely resembles the sedative-hypnotics in its behavioral effects. Potent *Cannabis* products (usually hashish) are not as frequently encountered within the United States, and, even when they are, they are normally used in very small quantities. It is only at high doses of THC that *Cannabis* resembles the psychedelics in its pharmacological effects. Thus, at least for the present discussion, THC will be classified as a unique psychoactive drug. In the future, as more is learned about brain function, THC may be more accurately classified. The structure of THC does not resemble that of any known or suspected chemical transmitters, and it is not known which transmitters in the brain are affected by THC.

HISTORICAL BACKGROUND

The history of *Cannabis sativa* from about 2700 B.C. until the nineteenth century still remains obscure. Marijuana was primarily used as a mild intoxicant, somewhat milder than alcohol and much less useful for religious and psychedelic experiences than the opiates or the naturally occuring psychedelics. Although products from *Cannabis sativa* were claimed to have a wide variety of medical uses, none of these uses seemed to persist for very long, and even today they have few documented medical uses.

Cannabis sativa is a rather new entry into Western culture. In the American colonies, the plant was widely grown in Virginia in the 1700s, presumably for its fiber, which was used for rope. Even George Washington grew hemp, presumably for its fiber, but possibly also for its medicinal and other properties. Hemp cultivation in the United States flourished for many years and then declined with the introduction of more profitable crops such as cotton and the importation of cheap hemp from the Far East. Periodically, however, hemp is still grown commercially in this country. During World War II, for example, cultivation was expanded in order to provide hemp when imports were severely limited. However, hemp need not be cultivated since *Cannabis sativa* grows wild and untended.

Marijuana, at least until the beginning of the twentieth century, was not widely used either in therapy or for recreation. This does not imply that psychoactive properties of marijuana had not been discovered (they had been), but they had not attracted the attention of the larger society, the use of marijuana being restricted to the "less desirable" element. In the early 1920s, the news media decided that marijuana was evil and was being used in the underground. In 1926, a New Orleans newspaper exposed the "menace of marijuana," claiming an association between marijuana and crime. Subsequently, laws were passed in Louisiana to outlaw the use of marijuana. Slowly, during the next five years, other newspapers took up the call, and more states began to pass laws against marijuana.

Probably the greatest impetus to the outlawing of marijuana was provided in the early 1930s by the Commissioner of Narcotics, Harry Anslinger, who had an intense interest in encouraging the states and the Bureau of Narcotics to enforce vigorously the laws against the drug. During the next few years, with the impetus of Mr. Anslinger, marijuana began to be looked upon as a narcotic, an agent responsible for crimes of violence, and a great danger to public safety. These attitudes were popularized through the 1930s by numerous news articles that served to convince the public that marijuana was indeed an evil. By approximately 1940, the country was convinced that marijuana was a "killer drug" and a potent narcotic that induced crimes of violence, led to heroin, destroyed the individual, and in general was one of the great menaces to society.

The campaign against marijuana and the emotion that it generated continued through the 1950s. The use of marijuana was still primarily restricted to the lower classes of society, for it was not often encountered by average citizens or their children. Then, in the late 1950s and early 1960s, marijuana and other psychoactive drugs became widely used by the middle- and upper-class youth. Through the 1960s, marijuana use by American youth increased steadily. Marijuana experimentation did not explode with the rapidity that LSD use rose, and the wide use of marijuana did not really develop until the later 1960s, when the use of LSD and other potent psychedelics had begun to decline. Marijuana then became more than a drug and was considered as a symbol of the younger generation.

It has been estimated that, by 1969, between 8 and 12 million Americans had smoked marijuana at least once.[1] A 1972 survey showed that more than 2 million Americans reported daily use of marijuana. A 1974 survey found that in one high-use county in California, 22 percent of the seventh-grade boys and 18 percent of seventh-grade girls reported having used marijuana at least once during the preceding year. A survey of 23-year-old men in 1974 found that 14 percent smoked marijuana daily during the preceding year. In this group, the daily use of marijuana exceeded the daily use of alcohol. Today the number of Americans who have smoked marijuana at least once may be close to 25 million.

ADMINISTRATION AND ABSORPTION

Most marijuana available in the United States has a THC content of approximately 1 percent, although the THC content varies tremendously and may range from near zero to as much as 3 or 4 percent. A similar range is found in marijuana from Southeast Asia. Marijuana grown in the United States usually has a THC content of less than 1 percent. The resin referred to as *hashish* (charas) usually has a THC content of anywhere from 5 to 12 percent. These figures will be important in the discussion of the pharmacological effects of *Cannabis* (next section).

In the United States, THC is usually administered in the form of a hand-rolled marijuana cigarette, the average cigarette containing between 1 and 2 grams of plant material. Thus, if a marijuana cigarette contained 1.5 grams of plant material with a THC content of 1 percent, the cigarette would contain approximately 0.015 gram (15 mg) of THC. Since THC is usually administered by smoking marijuana, the quantity of drug actually absorbed into the bloodstream varies considerably with the previous smoking experience of the user, the time the smoke is held in the lungs, the number of other users of the same cigarette, and so on.

Usually, individuals who have smoked marijuana several times can hold the smoke in their lungs for a longer period of time than can novices, therefore allowing a longer time for THC to be absorbed into the bloodstream before the smoke is exhaled. Similarly, individuals with a habit of inhaling the smoke of tobacco cigarettes usually can hold marijuana smoke in their lungs longer than can nonsmokers. The fewer individuals with whom the marijuana cigarette is shared, the more THC is available to each smoker. In general, approximately one-half of the THC present in a marijuana cigarette is actually available in the smoke. Thus, if a cigarette contained 15 mg of THC, about 7.5 mg would be available in the smoke. But it is extremely unlikely that one individual smoking one cigarette would be able to absorb 100 percent of the available THC in that cigarette. In practice, the amount of THC absorbed into the bloodstream from the social smoking of one cigarette is probably much less.

As we discussed in Chapter 1, the absorption of drugs that are inhaled through the lungs is rapid and complete. The onset of action of THC is usually within minutes after smoking begins and peak concentrations in plasma occur in from 10 to 30 minutes. Unless more is smoked, the effects seldom last longer than 2 or 3 hours. THC is also absorbed when administered orally, but the absorption is slow and incomplete. Administered orally, the onset of action is usually in 30 to 60 minutes, with peak effects occurring at 2 to 3 hours after ingestion. Effects persist for 3 to 5 hours or even longer. THC is approximately three times more effective when smoked than when taken orally. Since marijuana and hashish are crude preparations of plants and are not soluble in water, they should not be administered by injection. Indeed, injection of any crude product of *Cannabis sativa* or any other plant is extremely dangerous. It should be noted that what is sold on the street as "THC" is most frequently phencyclidine (see Chapter 8).

DISTRIBUTION, METABOLISM, AND EXCRETION

Since THC is only very slightly soluble in water, once it enters the bloodstream and is distributed to the various organs of the body, it tends to be deposited in the tissues, especially those that have significant concentrations of fatty material. Because THC is soluble in fat, it readily penetrates the brain; the blood-brain barrier does not appear to hinder its passage. THC may also be found in significant concentrations in the liver, kidneys, spleen, lungs, and even in the testes. Similarly, THC readily crosses the placental barrier and reaches the fetus. Unlike the opiates (Chapter 6), THC achieves levels in the brain comparable to those found in other tissues.

THC is almost completely metabolized to less active products before it is excreted. This metabolism is accomplished primarily in the liver but may also occur in other tissues, such as the lungs.

Unlike most of the psychoactive drugs that we have discussed, the metabolites of THC are excreted not only in the urine but also in the feces, in approximately equal proportions. In spite of being inhaled, THC is not excreted by the lungs as are volatile or gaseous anesthetics. The rates of metabolism and excretion of THC are rather slow. Approximately one-half is excreted within a few days, the rest usually within a week. Alcohol, by contrast, is metabolized and eliminated at a rate of approximately 10 ml of ethanol per hour. Some scientists feel that the excretion of the metabolites of THC may require more than one week and that some metabolites may persist for considerably longer periods. There is some evidence that some of the metabolites of THC are "active" and have relatively long durations of action.

PHARMACOLOGICAL EFFECTS

Within the last few years much information about the pharmacological effects of THC has become available. Research has been done on a variety of species, including mice, rats, cats, monkeys, and pigeons. Since many of these species differ markedly from humans one must consider the possibility of species differences and remember that people will not always react to a drug in the same manner as will an animal. However, if a drug produces similar effects in several species of animals, it is likely to exert similar effects in humans. If THC were to decrease behavioral activity in rats, mice, monkeys, and pigeons, it would probably do the same thing in people.

Effects on Animals

In almost all animal species, THC induces sedation and decreases both spontaneous motor activity and behavioral responses to painful stimuli. However, the doses usually employed in such experiments are high, usually between 5 and 20 mg of THC per kilogram (1 kg equals 2.2 pounds) of the animal's weight. This dose is between 200 and 800 times the dose usually administered to humans. In addition to this decrease in spontaneous motor activity, THC also decreases body temperature, calms aggressive behavior, potentiates the effects of barbiturates and other sedatives, blocks convulsions, depresses reflexes, and exerts other effects similar to those produced by the sedative-hypnotic compounds discussed in Chapter 3. In the monkey, THC produces sedation, decreases aggression, decreases the ability to perform complex behavioral tasks, and seems to induce hallucinations.

From studies in animals, one would conclude that THC, in its pharmacological effects, most closely resembles the sedative-hypnotic agents. It is presently not possible to examine in animals the psychedelic effects induced by THC, since we have no satisfactory way of studying hallucinations in an animal.

Effects on People

The commonly observed responses to either orally administered or smoked marijuana are seen as changes in the functioning of both the CNS and the cardiovascular system. Increases in pulse rate with a slightly decreased blood pressure are commonly encountered. Similarly, there is dilatation of the blood vessels of the cornea, resulting in the bloodshot eyes that are usually associated with indulgence in alcohol. THC users frequently report increased appetite, dry mouth, occasional dizziness, increased visual and auditory perception, and some nausea. Taste, touch, and smell may be enhanced. Time perception may be altered. Chronic smoking of marijuana has been associated with bronchitis and asthma. There appears to be some suppression of immune responses and possibly a decreased level of plasma testosterone (male hormone), although it is doubtful that these latter effects are any greater than those induced by alcohol or other sedative-hypnotic drugs. Driving performance is depressed.

Effects on the CNS are characterized by an increased sense of well-being, mild euphoria, feelings of relaxation, and relief from anxiety. All these effects, once again, resemble those induced by the sedative-hypnotic drugs. Higher doses of THC can induce delusions, feelings of paranoia, and hallucinations. There is confusion and disorientation, with altered sensory perception. Increasing anxiety may predominate. As doses are further increased, these drug effects intensify, with more vivid hallucinations, delusions, and increasing disorientation. However, since doses of this magnitude are seldom encountered in the United States, psychiatric emergencies as a result of smoking marijuana are extremely uncommon. Indeed, if one comes to an emergency room with a toxic psychosis purported to be due to "THC," the most likely drug of ingestion was phencyclidine, not THC.

THC also has mild analgesic properties, is a reasonably effective anticonvulsant, and decreases pressure of fluid within the eyes. Also, despite the fact that chronically smoked marijuana may induce asthma and bronchitis as side effects, THC decreases the resistance in the airways of the lung and therefore has potential therapeutic usefulness in the short-term treatment of asthma. These theoretical uses of marijuana as an analgesic, anticonvulsant, antiasthmatic, and agent useful in the treatment of glaucoma remained to be studied. Contrary to the opinion of many, marijuana is not an aphrodisiac.

While some side effects and long-term toxicities (see below) are now being recognized, it is clear that THC is a remarkably non-lethal compound. No deaths directly attributable to the use of preparations of marijuana have been reported. There is an extremely large safety margin between the recreational and the toxic or lethal doses of THC.

PSYCHOLOGICAL EFFECTS

In 1972, the National Committee on Marihuana and Drug Abuse reported:

> A description of an individual's feelings and state of consciousness as affected by low doses of marihuana is difficult; the condition is not similar to usual waking states and is the result of a highly individual experience. Perhaps the closest analogies are the experience of daydreaming or the moments just prior to falling asleep. . . . At low, usual "social" doses, the intoxicated individual may experience an increased sense of well-being: initial restlessness and hilarity followed by a dreamy, carefree state of relaxation; alteration of sensory perceptions including expansion of space and time; and a more vivid sense of touch, sight, smell, taste and sound; a feeling of hunger, especially a craving for sweets; and subtle changes in thought formation and expression. To an unknowing observer, an individual in this state of consciousness would not appear noticeably different from his normal state.[2]

Jaffe reported similarly:

> Most commonly there is an increased sense of well-being or euphoria, accompanied by feelings of relaxation or sleepiness when subjects are alone; where users can interact, sleepiness is less pronounced and there is often spontaneous laughter. . . . With oral doses of Δ^9-THC that are equivalent to several cigarettes, short-term memory is impaired and there is a deterioration in capacity to carry out tasks requiring multiple mental steps to reach a specific goal. This effect on memory-dependent, goal-directed behavior has been called "temporal disintegration," and is correlated with a tendency to confuse past, present, and future, and with depersonalization—a sense of strangeness and unreality about the self. . . . Although performance of relatively simple motor tasks and simple reaction times are relatively unimpaired until higher doses are reached, more complex tasks, such as those involved in driving, may be affected by doses equivalent to two cigarettes. Research subjects routinely report that they feel unable to drive while they feel "high" on oral doses of Δ^9-THC.[3]

Thus, the usual subjective effects of normal, social doses of marijuana consist of subtle mood alterations resembling daydreaming or mild sedative-hypnotic drug intoxication—alterations frequently imperceptible to the novice or the nonsmoking observer.

At higher doses of THC (several smoked marijuana cigarettes or moderate doses of hashish taken orally), the reactions mentioned above become intensified, but individuals are still in control of themselves and changes in their behavior would not usually be noticeable to an observer. Individuals experience intensification of emotional responses and alterations in sensation resembling mild sensory distortions or even mild hallucinations. In the current use of marijuana in the United States, such effects are seldom sought by the social smoker but more frequently by those few who use the drug to induce a pronounced state of sensory distortion.

With even higher doses (usually not seen in the United States, except in users of large amounts of hashish), one may experience extremely vivid hallucinations and psychedelic phenomena that include distortions in body image, loss of identity, sensory hallucinations, and fantasies similar to those induced by LSD, although less intense and probably more similar to the experiences induced by the milder psychedelic compounds such as mescaline.

Jaffe reports that these high-dose experiences induce frank hallucinations, delusions, and paranoid feelings. Thinking becomes confused and disorganized; depersonalization and altered time sense are accentuated. Anxiety reaching panic proportions may replace euphoria, often as a result of the feeling that the drug-induced state will never end. With high enough doses, the clinical picture is that of a toxic psychosis, with hallucinations, depersonalization, and loss of insight.[4]

Thought and motor activity are barely impaired at low, usual, social doses of THC but significantly impaired at higher doses. It is important to note, however, that the effects described above are normally achieved only with unusually large amounts of the drug, amounts that are more clearly related to the doses that decrease spontaneous motor activity in animals.

Thus, there are marked differences in the effects induced by usual social doses of marijuana and those induced by high doses of hashish. At social doses, effects consist of a mild sedative action most closely resembling a state of daydreaming. From this, one would tend to classify marijuana as a sedative, resembling alcohol or the other sedative-hypnotic agents. Marijuana, however, does not dull sensation as does alcohol but may induce mild alterations in perception. Whereas the sedative-hypnotic agents in high doses induce profound depression, coma, and even death, THC induces sensory alterations and hallucinations. At the usual low doses, there is little cognitive or motor dysfunction induced by the drug, but it may alter a person's ability to drive an automobile safely. Gross impairment of the ability to drive seems to occur only after high or extremely high doses of THC. Even then, such impairment may be less than that observed during alcohol intoxication. Nevertheless, driving while under the influence of marijuana should probably be discouraged, just as is driving while under the influence of alcohol. Moreover, the effects of marijuana and alcohol on driving are additive.[5] It has been demonstrated that smoking marijuana in socially used doses causes significant deterioration of simulated instrument flying ability in experienced pilots for at least two hours.[6] Therefore, acute marijuana intoxication is incompatible with the performance of complex tasks such as automobile or airplane operation.

SIDE EFFECTS AND TOXICITY

As we remarked above, THC is remarkably nonlethal, with perhaps the widest safety margin between recreational and lethal levels of any available psychoactive drug. Indeed, no verified deaths directly attributable to the use of *Cannabis* have been reported. The pharmacological effects of THC are so mild, consisting primarily of increased pulse rate and a reddening of the eyes, that physiological alterations induced by even heavy doses of the drug may not be perceptible either to the user or to a casual observer.

Although there are only minimal side effects associated with the *acute* use of marijuana, it now appears that *chronic* use of marijuana is associated with some degree of toxicity. Smoked marijuana has a definite bronchodilator effect and decreases airway resistance in the lungs,[7,8] but chronic smoking of marijuana and hashish is associated with the production of bronchitis and asthma, which presumably are due to inhalation as the route of drug administration. Clinical trials are currently underway to ascertain whether orally administered THC will be an effective antiasthmatic drug not associated with direct bronchial irritation.

In addition to the bronchial irritation, there is now evidence to indicate that long-term use of marijuana is associated with some degree of suppression of body immunity. The clinical significance of this effect is as yet unknown, although it should also be noted that other depressant drugs such as alcohol, barbiturates, benzodiazepines, and anticonvulsants share this immunosuppressive action.

Chronic use of marijuana has also been associated with reductions in the male hormone, testosterone. Although these data remain controversial,[9] this observation has been verified, and it can be preliminarily concluded that unrestricted marijuana use may lead to some reduction in testosterone levels[10] and possibly a reduced sperm count. It should be noted, however, that such depression of testosterone levels is also associated with the drinking of alcohol.[11]

Aside from the bronchitis (which is similar to that induced by cigarette smoking) and the reductions in body immunity and testosterone (similar to those induced by alcohol and other sedative-hypnotic drugs), there is little other evidence, to date, of any striking impairment of physical health or psychological functioning as a result of marijuana smoking. One persistent concern is loss of the work ethos and a possible loss of goal direction. Such concerns arose in the early 1970s with the observation of some American armed forces enlisted men using high doses of hashish on a chronic basis who exhibited apathy, dullness, impaired judgment, loss of interest in personal appearance, poor hygiene, and some loss of memory. Such effects were reversible with discontinuation of the drug. However, in two recent reports it was concluded that marijuana intoxication does not have any significant effect on motivation or on cognitive or psychomotor performance.[12,13] The National Commission on Marihuana and Drug Abuse concluded that "if heavy long-term marihuana use is linked to the formation of this complex of social, psychological and behavioral changes in young people, then it is only one of many contributing factors."[14]

There is at present no sound evidence to indicate that THC causes genetic abnormalities in humans, despite some reports of marijuana's decreasing litter size and growth rate in animals—effects produced only by extremely large doses that do not correspond to those used by humans.[15] It should be remembered, however, that THC (like all other psychoactive drugs) freely crosses the placental barrier and is distributed to the fetus. Therefore, as with the use of alcohol, cigarettes, and coffee, the smoking or ingestion of marijuana during pregnancy is to be questioned.

TOLERANCE AND DEPENDENCE

It appears that physical dependence on THC does not develop in animals or in humans even as a result of extremely high-dose, long-term use of the drug, and no significant withdrawal symptoms appear when the drug is no longer used. If dependence of any kind develops, it is most likely to be psychological in origin (rather than physiological) and even this appears to be only minimal. Only in extremely heavy users of THC does strong psychological dependence develop. Occasionally, minor withdrawal symptoms characteristic of psychological dependence may be observed. These include anxiety, restlessness, and other types of behavior similar to those observed in compulsive cigarette smokers.

With usual social doses of marijuana, tolerance (that is, a need to increase the dose in order to obtain the same effect) is not induced. In fact, marijuana may evoke a reverse tolerance: as a user learns how to appreciate the subtle alterations of mood induced by THC, it takes less and less marijuana to achieve a social high. Extremely high-dose, prolonged use of THC (such as that sometimes encountered in Far Eastern cultures) does result in some tolerance, and larger doses may be necessary to achieve a desired effect. As Szara states:

> I think it is justified to conclude at this point that the development of cannabis-type tolerance and physical dependence—as different from the opiate type—is a theoretical possibility, but its practical significance in a naturalistic setting—if any—is probably slight. . . . In conclusion, the results of studies presented in this volume [*The Pharmacology of Marihuana*] appear to justify the position taken by the *Fourth Marihuana and Health Report:* Occasional use may im-

pair perception, cognition, and driving ability but does not lead to detectable physical or mental health consequences. Everyday light use is already suspected of producing some deleterious effects and heavy daily use undoubtedly has some consequences in the function of pulmonary, hormonal, and central nervous systems. Exactly what these consequences are and how significant remain the subject of further extensive investigations.[16]

Indeed, in making a value judgment as to whether marijuana is good or bad, one is reminded of St. Thomas Aquinas, who said in *The Angelic Doctor* some 500 years ago: "Nothing is intrinsically good or evil, but its manner of usage may make it so."

MARIJUANA AND PUBLIC SAFETY

The first reports causally linking the use of marijuana to aggression, violence, and crime appeared during the 1930s. It was stated (with little factual basis) that marijuana led to antisocial acts, to crimes of violence and aggression, and even to the use of opiates.

As the Commission on Marihuana and Drug Abuse stated in 1972:

In the absence of adequate understanding of the effects of the drug, . . . largely unsubstantiated stories profoundly influenced public opinion and gave birth to the stereotype of the marihuana user as physically aggressive, lacking in self-control, irresponsible, mentally ill and, perhaps most alarming, criminally inclined and dangerous. . . . Now, more than 30 years later, many observers are skeptical about the existence of a cause-effect relationship between marijuana use and antisocial conduct.[17]

Major governmental reports written within the last few years are unanimous in their opinion that there is no scientific evidence that the use of marijuana itself is responsible for criminal behavior. There appears to be little or no relationship between marijuana and violent crime.[18] Marijuana is much less likely than alcohol to produce aggressive behavior. If there is any relation between drug use and crime, it is more likely that it results from the use of other psychoactive drugs that may produce aggressive behavior (such as alcohol or the amphetamines). As the National Commission on Marihuana and Drug Abuse pointed out:

In essence, neither informed current professional opinion nor empirical research, ranging from the 1930s to the present, has produced systematic evidence to support the thesis that marijuana use, by itself, either invariably or generally leads to or causes crime, including acts of violence, juvenile delinquency, or aggressive behavior. Instead the evidence suggests that sociolegal and cultural variables account for the apparent statistical correlation between marihuana use and crime or delinquency.[19]

The Commission concluded that

. . . neither the marihuana user nor the drug itself can be said to constitute a danger to public safety. For, as two researchers have so cogently stated for the Commission, "whatever an individual is, in all of his cultural, social, and psychological complexity, is not going to vanish in a puff of marihuana smoke!"[20]

CONCLUSIONS

After examining recent governmental surveys on the pharmacological and sociological effects of marijuana, we may conclude that marijuana, at least as it is currently used in this country, is the least potent of all psychoactive drugs in its effects on the body, on the brain, and on behavior. This is not to state that marijuana is a completely innocuous substance. Its active ingredient, THC, is still a drug that is freely distributed throughout all body compartments. Relatively speaking, however, marijuana has perhaps the greatest margin of safety of all available naturally occurring psychedelics and has been demonstrated to be of only minimal danger to the user.

The reader should keep in mind that THC is available in varying potencies. Hashish is an extract from *Cannabis sativa* and usually contains large amounts of THC. Marijuana is much lower in potency and, at normal doses, only a few milligrams of THC are absorbed into the bloodstream.

What, then, should be society's response to the known pharmacology of marijuana? Should the product be legalized and made available for widespread recreational use? Federal regulations under the Comprehensive Drug Abuse Prevention Control Act of 1970 provide the following penalties:

1. Cultivation, importation, and exportation of marijuana, and its sale or distribution for profit, are all felonies punishable by imprisonment for up to 5 years for the first offense and for up to 10 years for the second offense. (The penalty is double for sale to a minor.)

2. Possession of marijuana with intent to distribute it is a felony punishable by imprisonment for up to 5 years for the first offense and up to 10 years for a second offense.

3. Possession of marijuana for personal use is a misdemeanor punishable by up to one year in jail and a $1,000 fine for the first offense and up to two years in jail and a $2,000 fine for the second offense.

4. Transfer of a small amount of marijuana for no remuneration is a misdemeanor punishable by up to one year in jail and a $1,000 fine for the first offense and up to two years in jail and $2,000 fine for the second offense.

These federal regulations are meant only as a guide. In individual states, the penalties for possession or for casual exchange without remuneration can vary greatly. One of the first efforts should be to standardize state and federal legislation. If marijuana is a "dangerous drug," the greatest danger associated with smoking it may lie in being arrested and incarcerated. The pharmacological data presented in several government reports during the last few years and in studies dating back to 1894 indicate that the penalties imposed by the laws on marijuana may be far more serious than the "crime" that is committed by an individual's possessing small quantities of the drug.

There has been a wide range of opinion about the determination of social and legal policies dealing with marijuana. Over the years, however, those who have most closely studied marijuana (the India Hemp Drugs Commission, the La Guardia Committee, and the British, Canadian, and American commissions, to name a few) have all concluded that the individual and social risks associated with marijuana use are small. Recently the government has recommended that penalties for possession and use of small amounts of marijuana be liberalized.

Yet there are still some who, from reasonable observations, feel that the risks may be greater than we realize. Even these few individuals admit, however, that acute toxicities associated with marijuana use are unlikely. They caution, however, about a potential for toxicity when the product is used over long periods of time (one need only recall the toxicities just now being associated with long-term use of alcohol and tobacco). It may take one or two generations of users before this possibility is conclusively determined. However, in recent studies made in Jamaica and Greece, no significant tox- icities were observed to have developed even as a result of very long-term use of very large quantities of marijuana.[21] Professional and nonprofessional groups are agreed that marijuana possesses a low toxicity potential and that the likelihood of untoward, long-term tox- icity, though possible, is remote.

It is obvious that new legal policy must be formulated. As the National Commission on Marihuana and Drug Abuse reported in 1972, "The State is obliged to justify restraints on individual behav- ior."[22] Therefore, if the state is to maintain harsh marijuana laws, it should justify their severity. Present pharmacological data indicate that it may be difficult to justify arrest and incarceration for the use or possession of small amounts of marijuana.

Perhaps the most conservative course of action might be for society to maintain a policy of opposition to the widespread use of marijuana, as part of an attempt to discourage the use of *all* psycho- active drugs (at least insofar as they might endanger others), and refrain from punishing those who use marijuana (or at least mete out less severe punishment). Such a course of action was proposed by the National Commission on Marihuana and Drug Abuse, which recom- mended *only* the following changes in federal law:

—Possession of marijuana for personal use would no longer be an offense, but marijuana possessed in public would remain con- traband subject to summary seizure and forfeiture.

—Casual distribution of small amounts of marijuana for no remun- eration, or insignificant remuneration not involving profit, would no longer be an offense.[23]

The Commission further recommended that a plea of marijuana intox- ication shall not be a defense to any criminal act committed under its influence, nor shall proof of such intoxication constitute a negation of specific intent.[24]

These changes would essentially "decriminalize" the posses- sion of marijuana, and individuals apprehended with small quantities of the product would no longer be subject to a punishment that may be regarded as being more severe than the offense. The product would *not* be legalized, the state would continue to discourage its use, but those who possess marijuana would not be subject to punishment. Indeed, by August 1977, eight states (Alaska, California, Colorado, Maine, Minnesota, Ohio, Oregon, and South Dakota) had "de- criminalized" marijuana by removing felony penalties for simple possession of small amounts of the drug. Discussion of the effects of decriminalization in Oregon may be found in the paper by Blachly.[25]

In light of the known pharmacology of marijuana and its active ingredient, THC, repeal of prohibition is the most conservative change that society can make in its attitude toward *Cannabis*. However, Consumers Union went beyond the recommendations of the government reports and proposed the following:

> . . . the immediate repeal of all federal laws governing the growing, processing, transportation, sale, possession, and use of marihuana. . . . that each of the 50 states similarly repeal its existing marihuana laws and pass new laws legalizing the cultivation, processing, and orderly marketing of marihuana—subject to appropriate regulations. . . . an immediate end to imprisonment as a punishment for marihuana possession and for furnishing marihuana to friends. . . . [that] those now serving prison terms for possession of or sharing marihuana be set free, and that such marihuana offenses be expunged from all legal records.[26]

Consumers Union has thus taken a much more liberal position than the governments of Canada or the United States. That the recommendations will not be readily accepted was indicated by the National Commission on Marihuana and Drug Abuse in a second report in 1973:

> . . . the risk potential of marihuana is quite low compared to the potent psychoactive substances, and even its widespread consumption does not involve the social cost now associated with most of the stimulants and depressants. . . . Nonetheless, the Commission remains persuaded that availability of this drug should not be institutionalized at this time.

The commission's 1972 national survey data suggested that the incidence and prevalence of marijuana use might have peaked. However, a 1974 survey noted that marijuana use did not peak in 1972 but is still on the increase.[27] At the time of this writing, states that have not yet "decriminalized" marijuana possession are recognizing the reality of widespread marijuana use and are considering decriminalization. It is also becoming clear that there is little evidence to support the contention that marijuana use displaces the use of alcohol and other psychoactive drugs. Those who use marijuana are also likely to use alcohol, often simultaneously. The more heavily the user smokes marijuana, the greater the likelihood that he or she has used or will use other drugs. Such drug use may be related to a "drug-use proneness" and involvement with other drug users rather than to the characteristics of marijuana per se.

It appears, then, that society is adapting the position of accepting and tolerating (although not yet approving) the social use of marijuana as a recreational drug. Approval of marijuana for therapeutic purposes is under consideration but awaits proof of therapeutic efficacy.

NOTES

1. E. M. Brecher and *Consumer Reports* editors, *Licit and Illicit Drugs* (Mt. Vernon, N.Y.: Consumers Union, 1972), p. 430.

2. National Commission on Marihuana and Drug Abuse, Raymond P. Shafer, chairman, *Marihuana: A Signal of Misunderstanding* (New York: New American Library, 1972), p. 68.

3. J. H. Jaffe, "Drug Addiction and Drug Abuse," in *The Pharmacological Basis of Therapeutics,* 5th ed., L. S. Goodman and A. Gilman, eds. (New York: Macmillan, 1975), p. 306.

4. *Ibid.,* p. 307.

5. See M. Klonoff, *Science* 186 (25 October 1974): 317–24 and R. W. Hansteen, D. Miller, L. Lonero, L. D. Reid, and B. Jones, *Annals of the New York Academy of Sciences* 282 (1976): 240–56.

6. J. D. Blaine, N. P. Meacham, D. S. Janowsky, M. Schoor, and L. P. Bozzetti, "Marihuana Smoking in Simulated Flying Performance," in *The Pharmacology of Marihuana,* vol. 1, M. C. Braude and S. Szara, eds. (New York: Raven Press, 1976), pp. 445–47.

7. L. Vachon, P. Mikus, W. Morrissey, M. FitzGerald, and E. Gaensler, "Bronchial Effect of Marihuana Smoke in Asthma," in *The Pharmacology of Marihuana,* vol. 2, M. C. Braude and S. Szara, eds. (New York: Raven Press, 1976), pp. 777–84.

8. D. P. Dashkin, B. J. Schapario, and I. M. Frank, "Acute Effects of Marihuana on Airway Dynamics and Spontaneous and Experimentally Induced Bronchial Asthma," in *The Pharmacology of Marihuana,* vol. 2, M. C. Braude and S. Szara, eds. (New York: Raven Press, 1976), pp. 785–801.

9. See *Consumer Reports,* May 1975, pp. 143–49.

10. R. C. Kolodny, P. Lessin, G. Toro, W. H. Masters, and S. Cohen, "Depression of Plasma Testosterone with Acute Marihuana Administration," in *The Pharmacology of Marihuana,* vol. 1, M. C. Braude and S. Scara, eds. (New York: Raven Press, 1976), pp. 217–25.

11. G. G. Gordon, K. Altman, A. L. Southren, E. Rubin, and C. S. Lieber, "Effect of Alcohol (Ethanol) Administration on Sea-Hormone Metabolism in Normal Men," *New England Journal of Medicine* 295 (1976): 793–97.

12. P. J. Lessin and S. A. Thomas, "Assessment of the Chronic Effects of Marihuana on Motivation and Achievement: A Preliminary Report," in *The Pharmacology of Marihuana,* vol. 2, M. C. Braude and S. Szara, eds. (New York: Raven Press, 1976), pp. 681–83.

13. R. L. Dornbush, A. M. Freedman, and M. Fink, eds., "Chronic Cannabis Use," *Annals of the New York Academy of Sciences* 282 (1976): 1–57.

14. *Ibid.,* p. 76, fn. 7.

15. B. Mantilla-Plata and R. D. Harbison, "Influences of Alteration of Tetrahydrocannabinol Metabolism on Tetrahydro-Cannabinol-induced Teratogenesis," in *The Pharmacology of Marihuana,* vol. 2, M. C. Braude and S. Scara, eds. (New York: Raven Press, 1976), pp. 733–42.

16. S. Szara, in *The Pharmacology of Marihuana,* vol. 2, M. C. Braude and S. Szara, eds. (New York: Raven Press, 1976), p. 690.

17. National Commission on Marihuana and Drug Abuse, *Marihuana: A Signal of Misunderstanding,* p. 85.

18. J. R. Tinklenberg and P. Murphy, "Marihuana and Crime: A Survey Report," *Journal of Psychedelic Drugs* 5, no. 2 (1972), pp. 183–91.

19. National Commission on Marihuana and Drug Abuse, *Marihuana: A Signal of Misunderstanding,* p. 94.

20. *Ibid.,* p. 96.

21. *Ibid.,* pp. 76–81.

22. *Ibid.,* p. 159.

23. *Ibid.,* p. 191.

24. *Ibid.*

25. P. H. Blachly, "Effects of Decriminalization of Marijuana in Oregon," *Annals of the New York Academy of Sciences* 282 (1976): 405–15.

26. Brecher, *Licit and Illicit Drugs,* p. 535.

27. Secretary of Health, Education, and Welfare, *Marihuana and Health,* 4th Report to the U.S. Congress (Washington, D.C.: U.S. Government Printing Office, 1974).

Chapter 10

Birth Control and Fertility: How Drugs Modify Reproductive Systems

Although at first it might appear unusual, a chapter about the actions of the normal hormones of the body, especially those hormones used as contraceptives, is not out of place in a book about the effects of drugs that act on the nervous system and on neurons. Neurons interact with one another through the liberation of chemical transmitters, which are also called neurohormones (see Appendix II). The transmitters are liberated from one neuron, diffuse across a narrow synaptic cleft, and act on the postsynaptic membrane of the next neuron. These chemical transmitters are called neurohormones because, by definition, a hormone is a substance that is released by one cell and is then transported over some distance before exerting its effect upon a different organ or structure. The neurohormones are transported a very short distance from site of release to site of action

188

(in the range of 200 Å). The other normal hormones of the body (compounds such as the estrogens, insulin, thyroid hormone, growth hormone, testosterone, and so on) are released into the bloodstream and are transported in the blood to target organs that are some distance away (even several feet).

In addition to this physiological similarity between hormones and neurotransmitters, the brain exerts a regulatory role over the synthesis and release of both. For example, the estrogens are female hormones released from the ovaries but regulated by another hormone released from the hypothalamus, which has a receptor for the estrogens and is therefore sensitive to the levels of the estrogens in the blood. When estrogen levels are low, the hypothalamus releases a hormone that ultimately results in stimulation of the ovaries, which results in the production and release of estrogens. Birth-control pills, which contain a synthetically produced estrogen and a synthetically produced progesterone called a progestin, prevent conception largely as a result of the actions of the two drugs on these receptors in the hypothalamus. Thus, estrogens exert prominent effects on the hypothalamus and this "hormone feedback loop" is the mechanism through which the levels of estrogen in the body are regulated.

THE FEMALE REPRODUCTIVE SYSTEM AND HOW IT IS MODIFIED BY DRUGS

Figure 10.1 illustrates the principal organs of the human female reproductive system. These organs include the ovaries, the fallopian tubes, the uterus, and the vagina. The reproductive process involves the development of one ovum or several ova (eggs) in the ovaries. When it has developed in the ovary, a single ovum is released into the abdominal cavity. The ovum is not lost in the abdominal cavity because, in close proximity to the ovaries, extensions of the fallopian tubes called fimbriae (see Figure 10.1) gather the ovum into the opening of the fallopian tube, down which it is transported into the uterine cavity. If the ovum has been fertilized by a sperm (usually in its passage down the fallopian tube), it implants itself in the body of the uterus, where it develops into a fetus and a placenta.

The Monthly Ovarian Cycle

After puberty and the development of ovarian function, the normal sex life of a female is characterized by monthly rhythmic changes in the secretion of various sex hormones, together with cor-

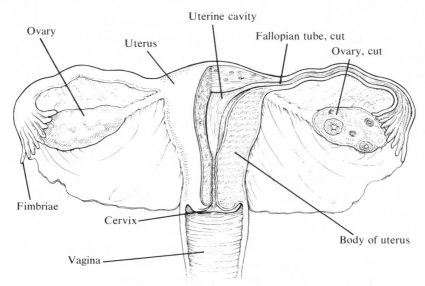

Figure 10.1. Principal organs of the female reproductive system.

responding changes in the activity of the female sexual organs themselves. The duration of this cycle averages 28 days but may vary from
20 days to as long as 45 days.

In order to accomplish the two most important aims of this
cycle—the development and release of a single ovum, and the prolif-
eration of a uterine endometrium that is prepared for the implantation
of a fertilized ovum—a coordinated sequence of hormonal events
must occur. This sequence of events is illustrated in Figure 10.2. At
the beginning of the cycle, the levels of both the estrogens and progesterone in the blood are low, the endometrium that was built up
during the preceding cycle begins to slough, and a several-day period
of menstruation occurs. Because these levels of estrogens and progesterone are low, the cells in the hypothalamus begin to release two
hormones: FSH-releasing factor (FSHRF) and LH-releasing factor
(LHRF). These two hormones are transported in the blood from the
hypothalamus to the pituitary gland, where they induce the release of
FSH (follicle-stimulating hormone) and LH (luteinizing hormone). In
response to the FSH in the blood, a variable number of ovarian
follicles (each containing an ovum) begin to enlarge. After five or six
days, one of these ovarian follicles begins to develop more rapidly
than the others, and the ovum begins to mature.

This maturing ovum then begins to release small quantities of
estrogens into the circulating blood. These estrogens act to inhibit the
further secretion of FSHRF from the hypothalamus and therefore to

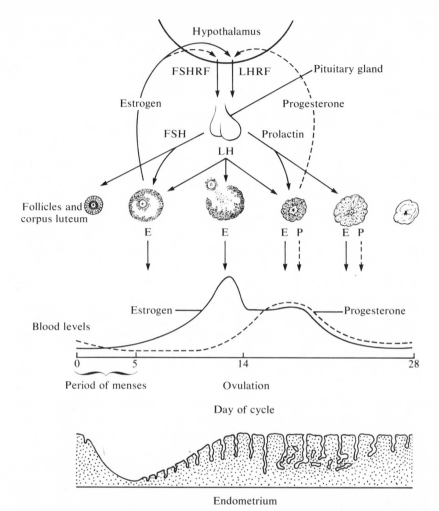

Figure 10.2. Sequence of events in brain, ovaries, and uterus during monthly ovarian cycle in female. *FSH,* follicle-stimulating hormone; *FSHRF,* FSH-releasing factor: *LH,* luteinizing hormone; *LHRF,* LH-releasing factor; *E,* estrogen; *P,* progesterone. *Solid arrows,* stimulation. *Dashed arrows,* inhibition.

inhibit the further release of FSH from the pituitary gland. This inhibition results in the regression of the other follicles that also had started to develop. The secretion of estrogens by the one maturing ovum and the follicle in which it is contained reaches a peak just before mid-cycle (day 14). Near the end of this preovulatory phase, LH is released from the pituitary gland under the stimulus of LHRF and prepares the ovarian follicle for ovulation by stimulating it to grow rapidly and swell to the point where it eventually ruptures and the developed ovum is released. This is referred to as the time of *ovulation*. LH is necessary for the final preovulatory development of the follicle and subsequent ovulation. Without LH (even with large quantities of FSH), the follicle will not rupture and ovulation is inhibited. (The pharmacological importance of this will be seen below.)

After ovulation, the ovum is gathered by the fimbriae into one of the fallopian tubes, where fertilization by a sperm is generally conceded to occur. The ovum (whether fertilized or not) then enters the uterine cavity. The follicle from which the ovum was released changes and becomes a structure called a *corpus luteum,* which secretes both progesterone and estrogens. These hormones released from the corpus luteum maintain the uterus in a state that is conducive to the receipt of a fertilized ovum. This is accomplished by the maintenance of a highly vascular endometrial lining (or endometrium) on the wall of the uterine body. In addition, the estrogens and progesterone released from the corpus luteum act on the hypothalamus to inhibit the release of FSHRF and LHRF. During the next 10 days, the corpus luteum regresses and within about 12 days ceases to function. Estrogens and progesterone being no longer released by the corpus luteum, menstruation begins and a new sexual cycle follows if fertilization did not occur. If the ovum were fertilized and implanted, the endometrium begins to secrete large quantities of hormones that act to maintain pregnancy and prevent menstrual sloughing.

Birth-Control Pills (Oral Contraceptives)

It has long been known that the administration of estrogens and progesterone, in sufficient doses, can inhibit ovulation. In 1957, Drs. Rock, Garcia, and Pincus demonstrated that ovulation could be prevented at will and for as long as desired by the administration of these agents.[1] The problem was to develop the appropriate combinations of estrogenic and progestational substances that would effectively suppress ovulation but would produce only minimal side effects with prolonged use. Excessive amounts of these substances might cause abnormal menstrual bleeding, while too little might fail to inhibit the release of FSHRF and LHRF from the hypothalamus, with the result being an unwanted pregnancy. Today, some 20 years since the introduction of these agents, we are still searching for the ideal oral contraceptive.

Speroff has recently reviewed this topic and he concludes that the low-dose combination pills, containing 30 μg of ethinyl estradiol, afford a reasonable compromise between toxicities produced by too much estrogen and bothersome breakthrough bleeding resulting from too little estrogen.[2] The three products currently available with 30 μg of ethinyl estradiol are Loestrin 1.5/30, Lo/Ovral and Zorane 1.5/30 (see Table 10.1).

COMBINATION OF ESTROGENS
AND PROGESTINS

By combining an estrogen and a progestin, release of both FSH and LH are blocked, ovarian follicles do not develop, and there is no ovulation. Two synthetic estrogens are used in the oral contraceptives. Natural estrogen cannot be used since it is not absorbed when administered orally. Adding an ethinyl group to estradiol (a natural estrogen) results in a compound that is orally absorbed. Thus, *ethinyl estradiol* is one commonly used estrogen. The second is *mestranol,* a compound that is converted in the body to ethinyl estradiol. While the estrogen inhibits the release of FSH, the progestin inhibits the release of LH, secondary to a block of release of LHRF. In addition to this action on the hypothalamus, the progestin acts on the uterus to produce an endometrium that is hostile to implantation of a fertilized ovum. The progestin also thickens the normal mucus discharge of the cervix so that sperm cannot gain access to the uterus and fallopian tubes (where fertilization occurs). All of these actions tend to decrease the likelihood of conception and implantation.

PROGESTATIONAL CONTRACEPTIVES

During the last few years, there has been increasing concern over the possibility that long-term use of the estrogens in the combination or the sequential oral contraceptives might be harmful. These fears have prompted the use of continuous progestational therapy without concomitant administration of estrogens.

As is apparent from Figure 10.2, if a progestational agent is given alone, FSH would still be released from the pituitary and an ovarian follicle would still mature. It is felt, however, that the progestin would greatly decrease the release of LH from the pituitary gland (secondary, of course, to a block of the release of LHRF from the hypothalamus) and the possibility of ovulations occurring would be slight. If, however, some LH were released from the pituitary, ovulation might not be completely blocked and an ovum would occasionally be released. Pregnancy would not necessarily result since the progestin also alters the structure and consistency of the endometrial

Table 10.1. Oral Contraceptives Available in the United States

Trade names	Manufacturer	Progestin	mg	Estrogen	μg
Brevicon	Syntex	norethindrone	0.5	ethinyl estradiol	35
Demulen	Searle	ethynodiol	1.0	–	50
Enovid-E	Searle	norethynodrel	2.5	ethinyl estradiol	100
Enovid-5	Searle	norethynodrel	5.0	mestranol	75
Loestrin-1/20	Parke-Davis	norethindrone	1.0	mestranol	20
Loestrin-1.5/30	Parke-Davis	norethindrone	1.5	mestranol	30
Lo/Ovral	Wyeth	norgestrel	0.3	ethinyl estradiol	30
Micronor	Ortho	norethindrone	0.35	ethinyl estradiol	30
Modicon	Ortho	norethindrone	0.50	–	35
Norinyl-1/50	Syntex	norethindrone	1.0	mestranol	50
Norinyl-1/80	Syntex	norethindrone	1.0	mestranol	50
Norinyl-2	Syntex	norethindrone	2.0	mestranol	100
Norlestrin-1/50	Parke-Davis	norethindrone	1.0	mestranol	50
Norlestrin-2.5	Parke-Davis	norethindrone	2.5	ethinyl estradiol	50
Nor-Q.D	Syntex	norethindrone	0.35	ethinyl estradiol	–
Ortho-Novum-1/50	Ortho	norethindrone	1.0	ethinyl estradiol	50
Ortho-Novum-1/80	Ortho	nonethindrone	1.0	–	80
Ortho-Novum-2	Ortho	norethindrone	2.0	mestranol	100
Ortho-Novum-10	Ortho	norethindrone	10.0	mestranol	60
Ovcon-35	Mead Johnson	norethindrone	0.4	ethinyl estradiol	35
Ovcon-50	Mead Johnson	norethindrone	1.0	ethinyl estradiol	50
Ovral	Wyeth	norgestrel	0.5	ethinyl estradiol	50
Ovrette	Wyeth	norgestrel	0.075	–	–
Ovulen	Searle	ethynodiol	1.0	mestranol	100
Zorane-1/20	Lederle	norethindrone	1.0	ethinyl estradiol	20
Zorane-1.5/30	Lederle	norethindrone	1.5	ethinyl estradiol	30
Zorane-1/50	Lederle	norethindrone	1.0	ethinyl estradiol	50

lining of the uterus and decreases the fluidity of the cervical mucus, which would restrict the passage of sperm into the fallopian tubes where fertilization usually occurs. Thus, although these agents consisting only of progestin *do not* totally block ovulation, they do tend to impede the sperm. Even if fertilization should occur, the progestin tends to prevent implantation of the fertilized ovum into the endometrium.

This discussion of *tendencies,* however, illustrates that the administration of a product consisting only of progestin (of which three are on the market at the time of this writing) is not quite as reliable as the administration of a combination product: statistics indicate an approximately threefold increase in the incidence of unwanted pregnancies. For women who experience significant side effects with combination products, administration of progestin only affords better contraceptive protection than is afforded by foams, creams, jellies, or rhythm and is certainly far better than no contraception at all.

Undesirable Effects of Estrogens and Progestins

The frequent, mild side effects induced by the contraceptive pill resemble those found in early pregnancy and are generally attributed to the estrogen in the combination or sequential products. These side effects are usually related to the dose, and products with less estrogen generally have milder side effects. These effects include nausea, occasional vomiting, headache, dizziness, weight gain, and discomfort in the breasts.

All may be alleviated if the woman is administered a product with *low* doses of estrogen (30 μg) or a product containing progestin only (Micronor, Nor-Q.D., or Ovrette). Breakthrough bleeding is a problem that appears to decrease with increasing doses of estrogen. As mentioned above, the products with 30 μg of estrogen offer virtually complete contraceptive protection, a minimum of serious side effects, and an acceptable level of breakthrough bleeding. If spotting or breakthrough is excessive, however, additional small amounts of ethinyl estradiol (20 μg daily for seven days) usually alleviate the problem.

Other side effects are generally not too bothersome and include weight gain and psychological changes that may result in depression in some individuals. These side effects are most frequently seen with the use of progestin-only pills or with the every three months (quarterly) injection of Depo-Medrol, a long-acting, injectable progestin.

Vaginal infections appear to be more common and more resistant to treatment in women who take oral contraceptives than in women who do not.

When administration of these agents is stopped, normal cyclic periods often are not immediately resumed, an effect that may prove a problem if a woman stops taking the pill in hopes of becoming pregnant immediately. It may take several months or possibly, for some women, one or two years to reestablish a normal cycle, presumably because the hypothalamus, pituitary gland, and ovaries have been suppressed for a prolonged time. However, approximately 95 percent of women whose menstrual periods were normal before taking oral contraceptives resume normal periods within a few months after cessation of the drug. Indeed, in those women who discontinue oral contraceptives to become pregnant, 50 percent conceive within three months and, more important, after two years only 7 to 15 percent have failed to conceive. Thus, there seems to be little or no increase in infertility in women discontinuing oral contraceptives.

Serious side effects observed with the use of oral contraceptives occur only infrequently. They include thrombophlebitis (the development of blood clots in the veins), pulmonary embolism (the lodging of a blood clot in the lungs), and cerebral thrombosis (the lodging of a blood clot in the brain). Current evidence indicates that the risk of death from these complications is about six times higher among users than among nonusers of birth-control pills (1.3 versus 0.2 deaths per 100,000 patients per year). However, the risk of death from all causes in pregnancy is 22.8 per 100,000 per year. Further discussion of the statistics involved may be found in the reviews by Speroff; Odell and Molitch;[3] and Murad and Gilman.[4]

It may be pointed out that even though the occurrence of these toxicities is statistically greater than that observed in women who are not pregnant and not taking the birth-control pills, they are usually conceded to be lower than those associated with pregnancy. This is not too surprising since the oral contraceptives essentially induce a state of pseudopregnancy—that is, the blood levels of estrogen and progesterone are elevated as they would be during normal pregnancy. Likewise, during normal pregnancy, the hypothalamus and pituitary gland are both inhibited by the same negative-feedback mechanism that is induced by the estrogens and progestins contained in birth-control pills. Because of this hormonal resemblance to normal pregnancy and the small associated risk of vascular disorders, many women feel that alternative forms of contraception, if feasible, may be desirable.

Other serious side effects that occur only infrequently but that may necessitate discontinuation of the drug include liver dysfunction (jaundice), emotional depression, increases in blood pressure, increased incidence of heart attacks, and increased risk of gall bladder disease. There is little evidence to indicate that oral contraceptives increase the likelihood of either breast cancer or cancer of the cervix.[5]

Because of the potential complications occasionally induced by oral contraceptives, strict controls have been placed on the labeling of these products. The Food and Drug Administration requires a statement that these compounds are not to be used where there may be suspicion of thrombophlebitis, danger of embolism, impairment of liver function, undiagnosed uterine bleeding, known or suspected pregnancy, known or suspected estrogen-dependent cancers, or known or suspected cancers of the breast. Since most of these complications are related to the estrogen in the product, it seems reasonable to use preparations with the lowest possible dose of estrogen; that is, in the range of 30 μg per tablet. In addition, it is extremely important to discuss with the physician the possible problems, toxicities, limitations, and alternatives to the use of oral contraceptives before use is initiated.

Alternatives to the Pill

Unfortunately, at present, there are few *effective* alternatives to birth-control pills when a woman desires to avoid pregnancy. At the moment, the most effective contraceptive practices include the pill, male or female sterilization, or abstention. Diaphragms, condoms, or intrauterine devices (IUD) are only approximately 90 to 95 percent effective. Even less effective are vaginal spermicides, the rhythm method, *coitus interruptus,* or douching. Thus, the most effective practices for *temporary* and *effective* prevention of unwanted pregnancy are the pill or abstention. Sterilization of either the male or female (although 100 percent effective) is *permanent* and should not be considered reversible.

Recently, estrogens administered in large doses have been used as postcoital contraceptives, particularly on college campuses.[6] The dose required for contraception is usually about 15 mg of diethylstilbesterol daily for several days. Apparently, the drug shortens the transit time of a fertilized ovum through the fallopian tube into the uterine cavity, which, for some reason, impairs the ability of the fertilized ovum to implant and survive in the endometrial lining of the uterus.

It has also been reported that single doses of progestins administered within three hours of intercourse can prevent pregnancy.[7] In a study of 2,801 patients who used this method of contraception for an average of 9.1 months and averaged eight coital experiences per month, the pregnancy rate was very low and side effects were mainly insignificant. Further study into this single-dose progestin method of contraception seems to be warranted.

More recently, a long-acting, injectable progestin administered at three-month intervals has proven to be an effective contraceptive.[8] The advantages of this form of contraceptive include freedom from daily tablet taking, freedom from the side effects of estrogens, and the maintenance of normal FSH activity. Disadvantages include breakthrough bleeding, weight gain, and depression.

Agents that Increase Fertility

Women who desire to conceive but may not be able to do so need a compound to *increase* fertility. Infertility may be the result of any of many factors (physical or psychological) in either the male or the female. Certainly the multiple causes of infertility cannot be discussed in detail in a book of this scope. Certain types of physical infertility in the female are susceptible to pharmacological manipulation. One such pharmacological approach is a direct extension of the scheme illustrated in Figure 10.2.

When estrogen acts upon the hypothalamus, the release of FSHRF is inhibited, the release of FSH by the pituitary gland is decreased, and follicular development is inhibited. If the action of estrogen on the hypothalamus were blocked, FSHRF would be released, and this would be followed by the release of FSH from the pituitary gland; subsequently, one or more ovarian follicles would develop and eventually at least one ovum would be released. For a drug to be capable of blocking the inhibitory action of estrogen on the hypothalamus, it would necessarily have to be capable of attaching to the normal estrogen receptors (thus blocking the normal access of estrogen to the receptor) and yet effect no change in cellular behavior.

Clomiphene (Clomid), a compound frequently referred to as a "fertility pill," is such a drug. Clomiphene has been responsible for conception by a large number of women who previously were unable to conceive. The drug has also been responsible for many multiple births; sometimes four or five ova are released and fertilized. The possibility of bearing more than one child is usually not a problem; frequently it is desired by couples who have not been able to conceive. Since clomiphene acts at the level of the hypothalamus, the pituitary gland and ovaries must be functional if the drug is to improve the chances of conception. The drug is ineffective when infertility is the result of a deficit in the male or when the female's infertility results from pituitary or ovarian dysfunction.

Ordinarily, clomiphene is taken starting on day 5 of the menstrual period (day 1 being the first day of menses), then taken daily for five days. The drug is stopped until the next menstrual cycle if the patient does not become pregnant. The procedure is then repeated, often with slowly increasing doses. A recent study indicates that approximately 35 percent of formerly infertile females became pregnant on clomiphene. Side effects of clomiphene include ovarian cysts (14 percent), multiple pregnancies (8 percent), and birth defects (2.4 percent). The incidence of birth defects in nontreated females is approximately 1 percent.

If a woman does not become pregnant after several trials on clomiphene, a newer compound called Pergonal (human postmenopausal hormone) is occasionally tried. Pergonal is FSH extracted from the urine of postmenopausal females. After menopause, since the ovaries do not secrete estrogen, the pituitary gland secretes large amounts of FSH. Pergonal is injected daily for 9 to 12 days, and after a day of rest an injection of progestin or LH is given. Approximately 75 percent of women so treated will ovulate, and approximately 25 percent become pregnant. Side effects of Pergonal include drug allergy, ovarian enlargement, blood clots, and occasional birth defects. At present, clomiphene is much more widely used than is Pergonal.

THE MALE REPRODUCTIVE SYSTEM

Figure 10.3 illustrates some of the important structures of the male reproductive system. The testes are situated within the scrotal sac and are composed of great numbers of seminiferous tubules in which sperm cells are formed. When formed, the sperm cells empty into the epididymus, where they are stored and mature. The epididymus leads into a long duct (the vas deferens) and the sperm cells are transported through this duct into the seminal vesicles and the prostate gland. In the upper vas deferens, they are mixed with fluids from both the prostate gland and the seminal vesicles. During ejacu-

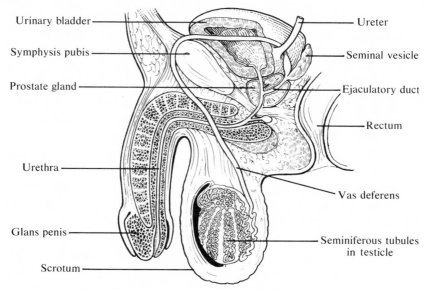

Figure 10.3. Principal organs of the male reproductive system.

lation, the prostate gland, the vas deferens, and the seminal vesicles all contract simultaneously so that the fluids and sperm cells are mixed and expelled through the ejaculatory duct and penis.

The actual neural control of arousal and of the male sexual act is extremely complicated, involving sensory input to the spinal cord and the brain and final coordination of motor activity to cause arousal with eventual ejaculation. The present discussion, however, is centered not so much on the act itself as on the hormonal regulation of the male reproductive system as a possible site of action of a male contraceptive.

If a drug could be developed to serve as a male contraceptive, it would most likely have to affect sperm production in the testes, sperm storage and maturation in the epididymus, sperm transport in the vas deferens, or the chemical constitution of the seminal fluid. All four processes are potentially susceptible to modification by drugs.

Hormonal Regulation of Male Fertility

The production of male sex hormones is closely controlled by hormones released by the hypothalamus and the pituitary gland (Figure 10.4). The most important male hormone is testosterone, which is formed in the testes by cells near the seminiferous tubules. The hormone is released into the bloodstream and distributed throughout the body. In general, testosterone is responsible for the distinguishing

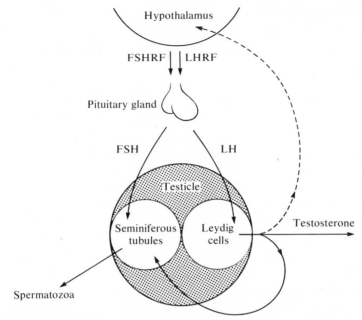

Figure 10.4. Hormonal regulation of male fertility. *Solid arrows,* stimulation. *Dashed arrows,* inhibition. (See legend for Figure 10.2 for explanation of abbreviations.) Note that the brain (hypothalamus and pituitary gland) is involved in the control of male fertility, just as it is in the control of female fertility. Note also, however, that fertility in the male is not subject to periodic cycling as it is in the female.

characteristics of the male: the development of male features including distribution of body hair, the lowering of voice, muscular development, bone growth, and other effects associated with the development of the male physique.

The production of testosterone is controlled by the hypothalamus. When testosterone levels in the blood decrease, LHRF is secreted from the hypothalamus and is carried in the blood to the pituitary gland, where it induces the release of LH, which then acts to promote the synthesis of testosterone in the testes. Testosterone in turn acts back on the hypothalamus to slow the rate of its own synthesis by blocking the release of LHRF.

The formation of sperm cells is controlled not by LHRF and LH but by FSH from the pituitary under the stimulus of FSHRF released from the hypothalamus. In the absence of FSH, sperm cells will not be produced. However, FSH alone will not cause complete sperm formation. Testosterone (secreted under the influence of LH) is also apparently necessary. Thus, both FSH and LH must be secreted by the pituitary if sperm cells are to be produced.

Male Contraceptives

In the search for a male contraceptive product, it would be convenient and efficient to interfere with sperm production by altering the hormonal cycle that involves the hypothalamus, pituitary gland, and testes; to be useful clinically, the drug would have to leave the LHRF-LH-testosterone system intact so as not to interfere with virility and libido. To date, no completely satisfactory product has been developed, although possibilities for the future are modestly bright. Products that *do* inhibit sperm production have been produced. However, all of them have induced side effects of sufficient intensity to limit their usefulness. Such side effects include the inhibition of the secretion of testosterone, with the resultant limitation of libido and virility. Since testosterone is necessary for the development of masculine characteristics, a drug that blocks testosterone synthesis would be undesirable. To date, no specific blocker of FSH activity has been developed. Similarly, no clinical acceptable drug has been found that alters sperm transport or viability.

The only currently effective contraceptive method in the male is vasectomy. At present this surgical technique, by which a portion of the vas deferens is removed, should be considered to be permanent and irreversible. It may be seen from Figure 10.3 that the cutting of the vas deferens would interfere only with the *transport* of sperm cells from the epididymus to the ejaculatory duct. Vasectomy does not interfere with masculinity, with sexual activity, with sperm production, or with the production of testosterone and therefore does not interfere with male virility, libido, or function. Fluids are still secreted from the prostate gland and seminal vesicles into the ejaculatory duct and, during the sexual act, fluid is still expelled upon ejaculation. It is only that this fluid does not contain sperm cells.

At present, the primary limitation to vasectomy is that it is irreversible. Perhaps, in the future a drug may still be found that would inhibit sperm production, storage, or transport or alter the properties of the seminal fluid so that the sperm cells would no longer be viable—contraceptive actions exerted in such a way that, when the use of the drug is discontinued, contraception would be reversible.

NOTES

1. J. Rock, C. M. Garcia, and G. Pincus, "Synthetic Progestins in the Normal Human Menstrual Cycle," *Recent Progress in Hormone Research* 13 (1957): 323–39.

2. L. Speroff, "Which Birth Control Pill Should Be Prescribed?" *Fertility and Sterility* 27 (1976): 997–1008.

3. W. D. Odell and M. E. Molitch, "The Pharmacology of Contraceptive Agents," in *Annual Review of Pharmacology*, vol. 14, H. W. Elliott, ed. (Palo Alto, Calif.: Annual Reviews, 1974), pp. 413–34.

4. F. Murad and A. G. Gilman, "Estrogens and Progestins," in *The Pharmacological Basis of Therapeutics*, 5th ed. L. S. Goodman and A. G. Gilman, eds. (New York: Macmillan, 1975), pp. 1423–50.

5. V. A. Drill, "Oral Contraceptives: Relation to Mammary Cancer, Benign Breast Lesions, and Cervical Cancer," in *Annual Review of Pharmacology*, vol. 15, H. W. Elliott, ed. (Palo Alto, Calif.: Annual Reviews, 1975), pp. 367–85.

6. Odell and Molitch, "The Pharmacology of Contraceptive Agents," p. 422, fn. 2.

7. *Ibid.*

8. *Ibid.*, pp. 1006–7, fn. 1.

Chapter 11

Drugs and Society: What Are the Alternatives?

The classic pharmacological approach to the communication of information about the actions of psychoactive drugs is to provide people with knowledge of the actions of these drugs—how the body absorbs, distributes, metabolizes, and excretes drugs; how the brain is organized and operates; how neuronal function is related to behavior; and finally how these functions are altered by psychoactive drugs. This approach avoids many complications inherent in an emotion-laden approach to education in the dangers of drugs and replaces it with an approach that takes the mystery out of drugs.

Of course, this approach provides explicit directions for people who are seeking to satisfy existing needs with drugs. This result has been amply demonstrated in education on drug abuse. Comprehensive education programs have frequently *increased* the extent of drug use rather than decrease it as was expected. However, the goal of drug education is not only to decrease drug use, but to provide accurate information, allowing people to make personal decisions about their own use of and attitudes toward drugs. Based upon such decisions, they can undertake examination and modification of risk-taking behavior.

THE OBJECTIVES OF DRUG EDUCATION

The approach used in this book was not taken with the goal of achieving an immediate impact on the use of drugs in our society. Education about drugs cannot achieve such a goal, and massive programs designed to eliminate or drastically reduce use of psychoactive drugs are likely doomed to failure. Society, either with or without drug education, will eventually learn about the effects of a given drug, but education may hasten this learning process and increase knowledge of the risk/benefit ratio that accompanies the use of any drug. Such knowledge will ultimately be disseminated into the community, and as a society learns of a drug's risks and benefits, a level of drug use (and abuse) that will depend upon this knowledge will become established. In short, it is hoped that, as a result of education, societies will be able to place drugs in their proper perspective. Education can function only to present the truth, as far as it is known. Indeed, although solid facts *can* be misinterpreted, they will serve society best in the long run.

This factual approach is also taken in hopes of countering much of the magic, mysticism, and emotionalism that is usually stirred up when one attempts to describe the effects of psychoactive drugs. In many social circles, discussion of psychoactive drugs evokes a very emotional response. It is hoped that by this method of presentation, discussion of the actions of psychoactive drugs will be concentrated on the drugs themselves as chemical entities and as compounds that alter processes in the brain.

Now that the pharmacology of psychoactive drugs has been presented, you should be able to compare and contrast the pharmacological effects induced by the different compounds. For example, there is presently controversy about the different effects induced by drinking alcohol or smoking marijuana. Chapters 4 and 9 should provide you with sufficient background so that you can compare the divergence of attitudes toward their use, a divergence that shows that people tend stoutly to defend their own pattern of drug use while condemning the use of different drugs by others. Several weekly news magazines have reported surveys of trends in drug use by young people and the response of parents to these shifting patterns of use. The magazines reported that the young people no longer tend to rely strictly upon marijuana as their primary psychoactive drug, they also adopt the drinking patterns of their parents. The parents were reported to be relieved that their children were no longer smoking marijuana but were now drinking alcohol. The pharmacology of these two drugs suggests we should question the wisdom of such a shift.

While many consider that such psychoactive drugs as marijuana, LSD, amphetamine, and the barbiturates carry some potential for toxicity, they overlook the fact that caffeine, nicotine, and alcohol are also psychoactive drugs with similar toxic potentials. Millions of people do not even consider these compounds to be drugs and, in many discussions of psychoactive drugs, these three are omitted. In chapters 4 and 5, the pharmacology and toxicity of these drugs were presented in detail and we noted that they all exert powerful effects on the brain, on the peripheral nervous system, on the heart, and on a variety of other body structures.

We noted the psychological dependence upon cigarettes, a dependence clearly illustrated by the inability of many individuals to abstain from smoking. We also noted the more serious toxicities associated with smoking: bronchial irritation, wheezing, chest pain, lung congestion, and lung cancer. We noted the toxic effects of smoking on the cardiovascular system: coronary heart disease, increases in heart rate and blood pressure, and possibly an increased predisposition to the formation of blood clots. We noted the effects on the developing fetus: increased rates of abortion, stillbirth, and early postpartum death in infants born of mothers who smoked during pregnancy.

If society is to become concerned about the recreational use of products containing drugs, it would seem, from the pharmacological and toxicological data, that the use of cigarettes should be discouraged. Certainly the efforts of many dedicated workers in the American Heart Association, the American Cancer Society, the Respiratory Diseases Association, and others are evidence of increasing public concern.

We should perhaps be similarly concerned about alcohol. As was illustrated in Chapter 4, alcohol is a sedative-hypnotic compound that, like all the sedatives, induces a state of behavioral disinhibition manifested by a variety of behavioral patterns that include euphoria, aggression, hostility, and altered driving behavior. Even though alcohol is considered by many not to be a drug, it is a powerful psychoactive agent that profoundly affects the behavior of the user and thus affects the social situation and social groups in which the user operates. Alcohol damages the brain, liver, pancreas, and other tissues to the extent of causing the deaths of 12,000 Americans a year. It is estimated that 50 percent of our highway deaths involve alcohol, and the drug is a factor in 70 percent of homicides. Currently, $10 billion are spent each year on alcohol by the 70 million users in this country, and about 7 million of these users are classified as alcoholics. Thus, along with public concern over the social use of marijuana, similar concern should also be directed toward cigarettes and alcohol.

Again, it should be the objective of drug education to increase the level of knowledge and awareness about the risk/benefit ratios of drugs so that meaningful comparisons between drugs can be made.

DRUG ABUSE

The term *drug abuse* is difficult to define. In general, it seems to imply the use of any drug for other than its assigned purposes. However, the concept of assigned purpose is vague. Does it refer to use only in medicine, or to use only according to a doctor's prescription? Does this mean that all uses of drugs for other than the treatment of medically diagnosed disorders is abuse of drugs? Are there no legitimate uses of drugs for recreational pursuits, for relaxation, for experience, or for temporary escape from reality? The history of man's use of psychoactive drugs (including alcohol) clearly indicates that there *is* such a role for psychoactive drugs and that it is not usually considered to be drug abuse. As our society becomes more crowded and more polluted, and as people become more frustrated and more angry, psychoactive drugs may become an acceptable form of recreation, relaxation, or escape, *in the absence of any better alternative*. The alternatives should be developed now, before psychoactive drugs do become the only course. Our experiences with alcohol pose a dim future for a society whose only form of escape becomes drug oriented.

Drug use, however, has been the prime recreational alternative for those whose geographical situation or economic status does not allow them enough room to live in. Drugs help one to tolerate confinement when one is unable to escape. When no other alternatives are available, drugs provide an effective means of altering one's mood or achieving altered states of consciousness, changes that are normal, not abnormal, human desires.

DRUG MISUSE

To avoid the emotion and imprecision of the term *drug abuse,* a new concept of the use of psychoactive drugs will be presented (see Table 11.1). This concept is not meant to replace the classification of psychoactive drugs presented in Chapter 2, by which drugs were classified according to their most prominent behavioral effect. It is intended to illustrate that legitimate uses of drugs are not all necessarily medical and that the use and the corresponding misuse of psychoactive drugs cannot be dictated by law. The concept accepts the obvious and recognizes that there are legitimate uses of drugs for recreation and as a means of experiencing altered states of consciousness. In Table 11.1, two broad categories of legitimate use of psychoactive drugs are proposed: medical and recreational. *Medically* legitimate are uses of psychoactive drugs in the treatment or prevention of diagnosed diseases or the alleviation of physical or mental discomfort. *Recreationally* legitimate are uses of drugs that generally involve the achievement of altered states of mood or of consciousness, relief from anxiety, induction of euphoria, or escape from uncomfortable or oppressive circumstances.

Drug misuse, then, may be described as the use of any drug (legal or illegal) for a medical or recreational purpose *when other alternatives are available, practical, or warranted, or where drug*

Table 11.1. The Medical and Recreational Uses of Psychoactive Drugs

Medical
  1. Treatment or prevention of diagnosed disease
  2. Alleviation of physical or mental discomfort

Recreational
  1. Relief from anxiety
  2. Achievement of a state of disinhibition or euphoria
  3. Achievement of altered states of consciousness
  4. Expansion of creative abilities
  5. Attempt to gain interpersonal or external insight
  6. Escape from uncomfortable or oppressive surroundings
  7. Experience of altered states of mood

use endangers either the users or others around them. In medicine, drug misuse would apply to the seeking, prescribing, or using of any drug for any purpose other than the prevention or treatment of diagnosed disease or the alleviation of physical or mental discomfort. A physician's prescribing a mild sedative-hypnotic tranquilizer for a patient merely because the patient requested the drug, or to terminate the interview with a patient, may be considered to be drug misuse. The misuse of a drug that may properly be used for recreational purposes occurs when the use of the drug impedes an individual's development outside the use of drugs, when it results in preoccupation with drug use, or when it endangers the physical or mental health of the individual or others.

ALTERNATIVES TO DRUGS

The concept of drug use presented in Table 11.1 leads to the final point of discussion in this book—namely, recognition of the fact that in order to combat drug misuse, *society must provide suitable alternatives.* Consider the following:

INTERVIEWER: Why do you use drugs?
USER: Why not?
INTERVIEWER: How could someone convince you to stop?
USER: Show me something better.[1]

This terse dialogue is incredibly significant. There is no way (the laws notwithstanding) in which we will stop either the recreational use or the medical misuse of drugs, especially psychoactive drugs, unless we provide suitable alternatives to the drug experience. As Dr. A. Y. Cohen states, drug use and misuse are widespread throughout our society:

> Even excluding alcohol, coffee, and cigarettes, it is now safe to estimate that over 50 percent of the total American population over 13 years of age has at least tried some powerful mind-altering drug via prescription or on the illicit market. Rare is the urban school using authentic survey data which reports that less than 50 percent of their secondary students have used amphetamines, psychedelics, barbiturates, cannabis products, and like drugs within the last twelve months. . . . In the adult world, one recent survey found that 25 percent of all American women over 30 were currently under prescription for amphetamines, barbiturates, or tranquilizers, the percentage going up to 40 percent for ladies of higher income families.[2]

Thus, it may be the exception rather than the rule for an individual to use no drugs at all. This is not to say that the use of psychoactive drugs is bad. What is clear is that use of psychoactive drugs for the purposes listed in Table 11.1 is widespread and will probably become even more widely accepted. Indeed, many segments of our society have accepted the concept of recreational pharmacology.

Recognizing this fact, recognizing the motives of persons who use drugs, and recognizing that it is basic human nature periodically to seek alterations in mood and altered states of consciousness, one can proceed to the active search for alternatives to drug use, alternatives that, if available, might reduce the incidence of drug misuse. As Cohen states, "Alternative is *not* just a synonym for 'substitute' since it implies an orientation which is *more effective* than drugs for giving the person real satisfaction."[3]

Numerous examples of alternatives could be presented. Table 11.2 is a listing of the types of experiences drug users might seek, their motives for seeking that experience, and possible alternatives that might help them attain that experience without drugs. (This table does not state that drugs should *not* be used to reach any of these levels of experience; it merely lists alternatives to drugs for those who desire alternatives that would allow them to reach particular levels of experience without having to resort to a pharmacological intermediary.)

The implementation of these alternatives should not be difficult. Brecher remarked that:

> . . . these and other "alternatives to the drug experience" are gaining favor among young people because they are superior to drugs, not because they are safer than drugs. An experienced drug user . . . "often finds that some form of meditation more effectively satisfies his desire to get high. One sees a great many drug takers give up drugs for meditation, but one does not see any meditators giving up meditation for drugs. Once you have learned from a drug what being high really is, you can begin to reproduce it without the drug; all persons who accomplish this feat testify that the nondrug high is superior."[4]

Further discussion of alternatives to drugs that may be used to achieve altered states of consciousness may be found in the report by Weil to the Ford Foundation.[5]

Table 11.2. Motives for, and Alternatives to, the Use of Drugs

Level of experience	Corresponding motives (examples)	Possible alternatives to drugs (examples)
Physical	Desire for physical satisfaction; physical relaxation; relief from sickness; desire for more energy; maintenance of physical dependency.	Athletics; dance; exercise; hiking; diet; health training; carpentry or outdoor work.
Sensory	Desire to stimulate sight, sound, touch, taste; need for sensual-sexual stimulation; desire to magnify sensorium.	Sensory awareness training; sky diving; experiencing sensory beauty of nature. [love making, swimming, running, mountaineering].
Emotional	Relief from psychological pain; attempt to solve personal perplexities; relief from bad mood; escape from anxiety; desire for emotional insight; liberation of feeling; emotional relaxation.	Competent individual counseling; well-run group therapy; instruction in psychology of personal development [sensitivity training].
Inter-personal	To gain peer acceptance; to break through interpersonal barriers; to "communicate," especially nonverbally; defiance of authority figures; cement two-person relationships, relaxation of interpersonal inhibition; solve interpersonal hangups.	Expertly managed sensitivity and encounter groups; well-run group therapy; instruction in social customs; confidence training; social-interpersonal counseling; emphasis on assisting others in distress via education; marriage.
Social (including socio-cultural and environ-mental)	To promote social change; to find identifiable subculture; to tune out intolerable environmental conditions, e.g., poverty; changing "awareness" of the "masses."	Social service; community action in positive social change; helping the poor, aged, infirm, young, tutoring handicapped; ecology action.
Political	To promote political change; identify with antiestablishment subgroup; to change drug legislation; out of desperation with the social-political order; to gain wealth or affluence or power.	Political service; political action, nonpartisan projects such as ecological lobbying; field work with politicians and public officials.

Table 11.2 (continued)

Level of experience	Corresponding motives (examples)	Possible alternatives to drugs (examples)
Intellectual	To escape mental boredom; out of intellectual curiosity; to solve cognitive problems; to gain new understanding in the world of ideas; to study better; to research one's own awareness; for science.	Intellectual excitement through reading; through discussion; creative games and puzzles; self-hypnosis; training in concentration; synectics— training in intellectual breakthroughs; memory training.
Creative-aesthetic	To improve creativity in the arts; to enhance enjoyment of art already produced, e.g., music; to enjoy imaginative mental productions.	Nongraded instruction in producing and/or appreciating art, music, drama, crafts, handiwork, cooking, sewing, gardening, writing, singing, etc.
Philo-sophical	To discover meaningful values; to grasp the nature of the universe; to find meaning in life; to help establish personal identity; to organize a belief structure.	Discussions, seminars, courses in the meaning of life; study of ethics, morality, the nature of reality; relevant philosophical literature; guided exploration of value systems.
Spiritual-mystical	To transcend orthodox religion; to develop spiritual insights; to reach higher levels of consciousness; to have Divine Visions; to communicate with God; to augment yogic practices; to get a spiritual shortcut; to attain enlightenment; to attain spiritual powers.	Exposure to nonchemical methods of spiritual development; study of world religions; introduction to applied mysticism, meditation; yogic techniques.
Miscella-neous	Adventure, risk, drama, "kicks," unexpressed motives; pro-drug general attitudes, etc.	"Outward Bound" survival training; combinations of alternatives above; pro-naturalness attitudes; brainwave training; meaningful employment, etc.

SOURCE: A. Y. Cohen, "The Journey Beyond Trips: Alternative to Drugs," in *It's So Good, Don't Even Try It Once: Heroin in Perspective*, D. E. Smith and G. R. Gay, eds. (Englewood Cliffs, N.J.: Prentice-Hall, 1972), pp. 191–92. Examples in brackets added.

NOTES

1. A. Y. Cohen, "The Journey Beyond Trips: Alternatives to Drugs," in *It's So Good, Don't Even Try It Once: Heroin in Perspective,* D. E. Smith and G. R. Gay, eds. (Englewood Cliffs, N.J.: Prentice-Hall, 1972), p. 186.

2. *Ibid.,* p. 187.

3. *Ibid.,* p. 189.

4. E. M. Brecher and *Consumers Reports* editors, *Licit and Illicit Drugs* (Mt. Vernon, N.Y.: Consumers Union, 1972), p. 510.

5. A. T. Weil, "Altered States of Consciousness," in *Dealing with Drug Abuse* (a report to the Ford Foundation), Drug Abuse Survey Project, P. M. Wald and P. B. Hutt, cochairmen (New York: Praeger, 1972).

The Physiology of the Nerve Cell

In studying the nervous system, it soon becomes apparent that structure and function are so clearly related that, before function may be discussed, one must possess some knowledge of structure. In addition, if one is to discuss the effects of drugs on the nervous system, it is helpful to have grasped the principles of the structure and function of the basic element of the nervous system, namely, the *nerve cell (the neuron)*.

Nerve cells exhibit two special properties that distinguish them from all other cells of the body. The first is their ability to conduct electrical impulses over long distances. The second is that they have specific input and output relationships both with other nerve cells and with other tissues of the body whose functions the neurons may control (such as muscles and glands). These input-output connections determine the function of the particular neuron and, in turn, the patterns of response that the neuron may elicit.

THE BRAIN

The human brain comprises some 13 billion neurons. Most of them share common structural and functional characteristics. Structurally, the typical neuron consists of a cell body that contains the nucleus of the cell and is often referred to as the *soma*. Extending out from the soma are many short fibers called *dendrites,* which respond to the electrical activity of other neurons and which conduct such activity to the soma. Also extending from the soma is a fiber called the *axon,* which may be either short or up to 3 feet long (as are the axons projecting down the spinal cord or running from the spinal cord to the muscles). The axon transmits activity from the soma to other neurons or to the muscles or glands of the body. In general, the axon conducts impulses in only one direction: from the soma down the axon to a specialized terminal called the *synapse.* At the synapse, a chemical (the transmitter substance) is released and diffuses across a gap, the synaptic cleft, to the dendrite of the next neuron, thereby

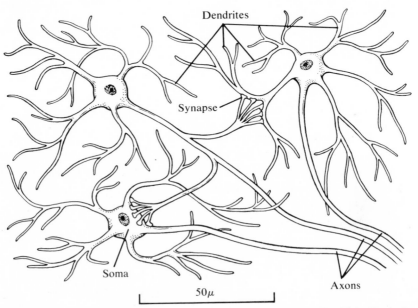

Figure I.1. Schematic representation of three nerve cells. This illustrates the major subdivisions of such cells and the interactions between them.

transmitting information from one neuron to another. The neurons do not physically touch each other.

Figure I.1 illustrates three neurons and their interactions with one another. Figure I.2 is an illustration of more typical neuronal interactions. Usually, only one axon will arise from the soma, but in its projection, the axon may give off many side branches, sending impulses to a great number of other neurons (causing a divergence of information). Several dendrites arise from one soma. These dendrites branch profusely to form a complex structure sometimes referred to as a *dendritic tree*. This dendritic network receives as many as 50,000 contacts from other cells (resulting in the convergence of information), processes the impulses, and transmits electrical activity to the soma. The soma in turn transmits the impulses it received from the dendrites to as many as 10,000 other neurons. Thus, a great many neurons converge on one neuron, which in turn spreads its own impulses to many other neurons. Most cells elsewhere in the body function as isolated entities; neurons are interconnected in specific manners.

As a consequence of this convergence and divergence of electrical activity, neurons tend to group together and form circuits, and it is the properties of these circuits that determine the way in which

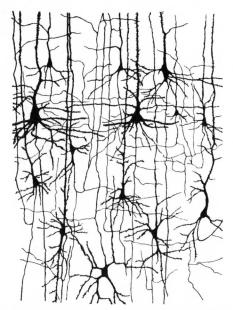

Figure I.2. Diagrammatic representation of neuronal architecture in the cerebral cortex. [From S. Ramón y Cajal, 1900–1906.]

information is handled in the nervous system and thus the behavior of the animal. These neural circuits will be discussed in detail in Appendix III. As an overview, however, it can be stated that it is possible to distinguish those areas of the brain where cell bodies and their dendrites are concentrated (these areas are referred to as *nuclei*) from those regions that consist mainly of the axons projecting from one group of neurons to another (these regions are referred to as *fiber tracts*). Thus, axons are sometimes called *fibers* or *nerve fibers*. In the peripheral nervous system (that is, outside the brain and spinal cord), bundles of these axons are commonly referred to as *nerves*.

In the brain, the somas of several thousand neurons group together to form structures called *nuclei*. (Further, these nuclei tend to congregate to form yet larger structures, such as the thalamus, hypothalamus, amygdala, and hippocampus.) Each nucleus consists of tens of thousands of individual nerve-cell bodies (somas). The fiber tracts of the brain are often given names indicating the areas of the brain connected by the tracts. For instance, the bundle of axons running from the cortex to the thalamus is referred to as the cortico-thalamic tract.

In addition to the nerve cells, many other types of cells are found in the brain. The most conspicuous of these are the *glial cells,* one type of which (the astrocyte) we discussed as surrounding the brain capillaries to form part of the blood-brain barrier. Other glial cells provide structural support for the brain or metabolic support for the neurons in an as yet unidentified fashion.

In summary, one neurophysiology text describes the brain as follows:

> The brain, then, is an immense number of spidery nerve cells, interconnected in a complex net, and embedded in a supporting and protecting meshwork of neuroglia. Dendrites spring from the neuron cell body, branch profusely, and along with the soma receive myriads of axon terminals, making it possible for a single nerve cell to gather information from hundreds of others. Furthermore, cell bodies are collected into groups, the nuclei, and these in turn into clusters. Running back and forth between nuclei or between collections of nuclei are fiber tracts, the main channels of communications between one part of the brain and another. Altogether, these structures are arranged in an orderly way to form the brain of the animal and to provide the anatomical basis for neural function.[1]

Psychoactive drugs exert their behavioral effects secondary to alterations in the specific channels of information in specific areas of the brain.

THE AXON

The neuron is the primary element of the nervous system and consists of three main divisions: the dendrites, the soma, and the axon. In brief, electrical impulses originate in the dendrites, are integrated in the soma (where the action potentials are formed), and are transmitted down the axon to the synapse. Unlike the dendrites and the soma, the axon is the part of the cell that is specialized *solely* for the rapid and reliable conduction of electrical activity, in the form of electrical impulses called *action potentials*. All action potentials conducted down a given axon are essentially identical, and the only manner in which changes in content can be relayed by the axon is by alterations in the number of action potentials conducted each second.

The axon is, in general, not a major site of action of psychoactive drugs, but it is the site of action of some important drugs, foremost of which are the local anesthetics. Lidocaine (Xylocaine), for example, is a local anesthetic that, when injected into the tissues surrounding the sensory nerves from a tooth, effectively blocks transmission of pain impulses that travel from the nerve endings (specialized dendrites) in the tooth to the brain. The anesthetic does not directly affect the tooth but only blocks the axons in the nerve trunks that are carrying information to the brain.

Most psychoactive drugs exert their effects not on the axon but at the synaptic junction between the axon of one cell and dendrites of another. However, since local anesthetics affect the axon and since the axon is essential for the conduction of action potentials, the properties and functions of the axon are discussed further at the end of this appendix.

THE DENDRITES

The axon, which specializes in the transmission of action potentials from the soma to the synapse, has the ability to conduct electrical impulses over its full length rapidly and without alteration. Thus, to this point, we have impulses traveling down an axon to the synapse, the functional junction between two separate neurons. How are these impulses then transmitted to the next neuron? In brief, the terminals of the axon align themselves at the synapse in close approximation to the dendrites of the next neuron (Figure I.1). It is this site of connection between the axon terminal and the dendrite that is the point at which impulses are transferred between neurons in the nervous system (see Appendix II).

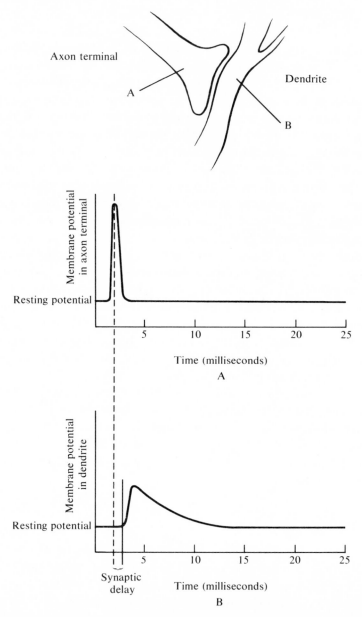

Figure I.3. Transmission of impulses from one neuron to another at a synapse. Graph *A* is a recording of electrical activity in the axon terminal as an action potential arrives at the synapse. Graph *B* is a recording of electrical activity in the dendrite of the next neuron showing the postsynaptic activity resulting from the transmission of impulses across the synapse. [Modified from C. F. Stevens, *Neurophysiology: A Primer* (New York: John Wiley, 1966), fig. 3-2, p. 35.]

The dendrites are structures specialized for the receipt of impulses from other neurons. When action potentials have been conducted down the axon of one neuron, the dendrite with which the axon synapses exhibits an electrical change, the magnitude of which is directly proportional to the frequency at which impulses arrive from the axon (Figure I.3). When the impulses arrive at the synapse, a chemical transmitter is released, diffuses across a small, fluid-filled gap (the synaptic cleft), and alters the dendritic membrane. If the transmitter chemical affects the membrane in such a manner that the membrane depolarizes, the neuron becomes more excitable (Figure I.3). This depolarization is referred to by physiologists as an *excitatory postsynaptic potential* (EPSP). Note from Figure I.3 that there is a slight delay (approximately 0.5 milliseconds) between the arrival of the action potential at the nerve terminal and the EPSP in the dendritic membrane. This time lag is called the *synaptic delay* and is explained by the time required for the transmitter substance released by the axon to reach the dendrite of the next cell. Thus, cells in the brain are connected with one another chemically rather than electrically or physically. The synapse is the prime site of action of most psychoactive drugs.

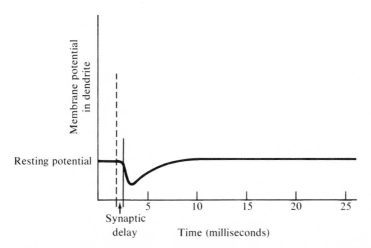

Figure I.4. An inhibitory postsynaptic potential. Recorded from the dendrite of a neuron that has received impulses across an inhibitory synapse—that is, the chemical transmitter liberated by the presynaptic nerve terminal is inhibitory to the postsynaptic membrane. The nerve impulse arrived at the axon terminal of the presynaptic neuron at the time indicated by the arrow. [Modified from C. F. Stevens, *Neurophysiology: A Primer* (New York: John Wiley, 1966), fig. 3-9, p. 44.]

Thus, the axon is electrically excitable and capable of conducting action potentials rapidly. The dendrite is chemically excitable (by transmitter) and, if the membrane is depolarized, excitatory postsynaptic potentials are induced.

In the central nervous system, all neurons are held in a balance between excitation and inhibition. If *all* synapses were excitatory, we would convulse continuously, since every cell in the brain would be discharging at an uncontrolled rate. In order to balance excitation, there must be a process of inhibition. Some transmitter chemicals, instead of depolarizing the dendrites, induce a *hyperpolarization* of the dendritic membrane (Figure I.4). This hyperpolarizing potential is referred to as an inhibitory postsynaptic potential (IPSP). This IPSP opposes the action of EPSPs, stabilizes the neuron, and tends to prevent the generation of action potentials.

Thus, although only one type of action potential may be carried down an axon, two types of chemical transmitters can be released, depending upon the neuron: transmitters that depolarize the dendritic membrane or those that hyperpolarize it. All cells in the nervous system receive impulses from both excitatory and inhibitory synapses. Indeed, the exquisite beauty of the nervous system is maintained by this delicate balance between excitation and inhibition.

The dendrites of a single nerve cell may make as many as 50,000 synapses with axons from other cells. The influence of an individual synaptic connection may be excitatory or inhibitory, and the type of activity seen in the postsynaptic neuron will depend upon the influence exerted by the preponderance of presynaptic neurons. Psychoactive drugs, since they affect synaptic transmission, tend to upset this balance of excitation and inhibition. It is the result of this alteration of excitability within specific areas of the nervous system that leads to drug-induced alterations in behavior.

THE SOMA

The dendrite receives input from other neurons through the synapses and responds by either depolarizing (increasing excitability) or hyperpolarizing (decreasing excitability). All of the impulses received at the dendrites affects the level of excitability of the soma (the cell body), which gives rise to only a single axon and thus to a single channel through which these impulses are transmitted to other neurons. How, then, are the electrical potentials from the dendrites converted into an action potential? It appears that the soma integrates (or averages) the impulses gathered by the dendrites. If the influence of excitatory synapses is sufficiently greater than the influence of inhibitory synapses, the soma will respond by producing an action potential that spreads into the axon and is conducted to the next synapse. If more inhibitory input is received than excitatory input, the soma will hyperpolarize and the neuron will become less excitable. The soma, therefore, expresses the integration of the dendritic input as depolarization or hyperpolarization (depolarization resulting in the generation of an action potential and hyperpolarization resulting in the blockage of the generation of an action potential).

Concerning the actions of drugs, we have stated that the psychoactive drugs exert their behavioral effects by altering the delicate balance of excitation and inhibition generated by the processes of synaptic transmission.

PROPERTIES OF EXCITABLE MEMBRANES

All fluid outside the bloodstream is either inside cellular membranes (intracellular fluid) or outside the cells, surrounding them but remaining outside the bloodstream (extracellular fluid). An important difference between extracellular and intracellular fluid is the marked imbalance in the concentration of certain ions (small, electrically charged molecules), which results largely from the varying permeability of the cell membrane to water-soluble, fat-insoluble substances. The cell membranes are structures of protein and fat containing small, water-filled pores. These pores are about 7 Å in diameter. The movement of substances through these pores is limited by the size of pores. Because of the size of the pores, the membrane is freely permeable to potassium ions (K^+) and chloride ions (Cl^-), which are smaller than 7 Å; relatively impermeable to sodium ions (Na^+); and essentially impermeable to organic anions (A^-), which are present as large protein molecules. The concentrations of sodium (Na^+) and chloride (Cl^-) are much higher in the extracellular fluid than in the intracellular fluid, and the concentrations of potassium (K^+) and organic anions (A^-) are much higher in the intracellular fluid than in the extracellular fluid. These differences of concentration are illustrated in Figure I.5.

As a consequence of this ionic imbalance on either side of the cell membrane, there is an electrical potential (difference in voltage)

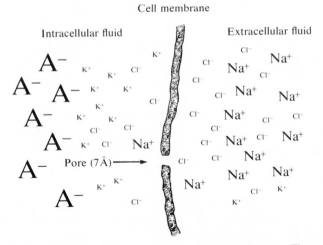

Cell membrane

Intracellular fluid

Extracellular fluid

Figure I.5. Distribution of ions across a cell membrane. The cell membrane is a protein-fat barrier (see Figure 1.3) that apparently contains small pores, approximately 7 Å in diameter, that allow the passage of water and of certain small ions. Na^+, sodium ions; Cl^-, chloride ions; K^+, potassium ions; A^-, large protein molecules that contain negative charges. As their relative sizes indicate, potassium and chloride ions are able to diffuse freely through the pores, while sodium ions are less able to do so and protein molecules are largely not able to diffuse.

across the membrane. This electrical potential may reach 50 to 90 millivolts, with the inside negative in relation to the outside. Such difference in potential exists in every cell of the body (not only neurons) and is referred to as the *resting potential* of the cell, although the magnitude of the resting potential varies from cell type to cell type. Positive charges tend to move into the cell, and negative charges tend to move out. However, sodium ions (which are positive and are to be found in high concentrations outside the cell) penetrate the membrane very poorly, and the negatively charged organic proteins (A^-) on the interior of the cell are unable to move out. Such distribution of ions keeps the electrical charges distant from each other and thus maintains the resting potential.

Since *all* cells of the body exhibit this resting potential, what distinguishes nerve cells (which are excitable structures capable of generating action potentials) from all other cells of the body? When the neuron becomes less negative (in relation to extracellular fluid) the axon is said to be depolarized (Figure I.6). When the axon is depolarized by a few millivolts, the permeability of the membrane is altered so that the membrane becomes rapidly more permeable to Na^+. Within a fraction of a millisecond, sodium ions traverse the

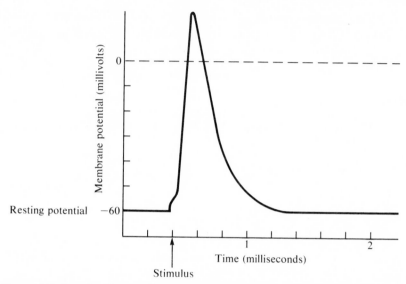

Figure I.6. Graph of an action potential. Stimulus was applied at the time indicated by the arrow. [From C. F. Stevens, *Neurophysiology: A Primer* (New York: John Wiley, 1966), fig. 2-3, p. 14.]

membrane from the outside to the inside of the cell, neutralizing the electrical potential that was formerly maintained across the membrane. So many sodium ions enter the neuron, in fact, that the membrane potential slightly overshoots the neutral potential (0) and the inside of the cell becomes slightly positive in relation to the outside. At this point, the membrane loses its increased permeability to sodium ions, no more enter, and potassium ions (which are in high concentrations on the inside of the cell, and which can easily traverse the membrane) leave the cell to restore the difference in potential. Thus, the cell has gone through a brief period during which it has had its resting state upset, and become slightly positive on the inside. Through a "pump," the membrane redistributes the ions and restores the original resting potential. All these events, which occur within a period of about one one-thousandth of a second, constitute a sequence called an *action potential*.

In addition to electrical excitability, the axon exhibits another important characteristic: the ability to conduct the action potential the length of the axon without alteration or decrease in intensity. (The mechanisms by which the ionic gradients are maintained and reestablished after excitation are complicated and beyond the scope of the present discussion. Discussions of these topics may be found in the readings listed in the bibliography.)

The axon is capable of conducting impulses at widely varying frequencies, from less than one per second to as much as 500 per second, depending upon the degree of depolarization of the soma.

NOTE

1. C. F. Stevens, *Neurophysiology: A Primer* (New York: John Wiley, 1966), p. 8.

Synaptic Transmission and Transmitters

In Appendix I we discussed the electrical phenomena that characterize neurons as unique entities and that are the basis of nervous-system function. We explained that all information transfer in the brain is accomplished by the interaction of neurons with one another. We discussed the dendrite as the recipient of chemical transmitters released by other neurons, the soma as the integrator, and the axon as the structure that transmits action potentials to the synapse. Chemicals released at the synapse then influence the activity of other neurons. We said nothing, however, about how impulses are transmitted from one neuron to another or from neurons to effector organs (muscles or gland cells).

There is now almost universal acceptance of the theory of chemical transmission between neurons. This merely means that transmission across synapses occurs by means of specific agents referred to as *chemical transmitters*. As will be seen, the actions of most psychoactive drugs can be interpreted in terms of their mimicking or modifying the actions of these transmitters. This concept of chemical transmission between neurons holds that action potentials conducted down an axon cause the release of specific chemical substances when these potentials reach the axon terminal. These chemicals are, in turn, capable of altering the permeability of the dendritic membrane of the next neuron, resulting in either a depolarization (EPSP) or hyperpolarization (IPSP) of the dendrites of that neuron.

We shall now discuss the steps involved in synaptic transmission and the criteria that a chemical must meet in order to be called a transmitter substance. We shall also discuss specific substances that are thought to function in the central nervous system as synaptic transmitters.

HISTORICAL BACKGROUND

The first suggestion that chemical substances might be involved in the transmission of information between neurons was probably made by DuBois-Reymond in 1877. Subsequent work by physiologists such as Langley (1901), Elliot (1904), Dixon (1907), and Dale (1914) established the foundation for the concept that "excitation of a nerve induces the local liberation of a hormone, which causes specific activity by combination with some constituent of the end-organ, muscle or gland." From the work of these early physiologists came later the identification of acetylcholine and epinephrine as transmitter substances in the peripheral nervous system (nerves lying outside the brain and spinal cord).

In 1921, Otto Loewi presented the first definite proof for the chemical mediation of nerve-impulse transmission. Loewi took the hearts out of two frogs and suspended the hearts from a frame. Because the rate at which a heart beats is controlled by nerve fibers (axons) that lead to the heart from the brain, Loewi electrically stimulated the nerve leading to one of the two hearts. He found that such stimulation slowed the rate at which the heart beat. Loewi dripped fluid over the heart that he was stimulating, then took this fluid and dripped it over the second heart (which was not being stimulated); he found that its rate also became slower. This demonstrated that electrical stimulation of the nerve leading to the one heart caused the release of a chemical that could slow the rate of the other heart, the nerves of which were not stimulated, proving that nerves exert their effects by releasing chemicals that act on the structure that the nerves innervate.

Loewi subsequently identified this substance as acetylcholine. He later also discovered that a chemical substance similar to epinephrine was liberated when the accelerator nerve to the heart was stimulated. Epinephrine is a transmitter substance important in the maintenance of many body functions, including heart rate, blood pressure, pupil size, lung function, and sex drive. Since these experiments were performed in cold-blooded animals (frogs), the experiments were repeated in 1927 by Rylant in the perfused rabbit heart. These and other investigations through the 1930s and 1940s established quite conclusively that a chemical mediator is instrumental in the transmission of impulses across synapses. Finally, in 1946 Euler identified norepinephrine as the chemical transmitter in the peripheral sympathetic nervous system. These early developments in studies of neurohumoral transmission are well detailed by Koelle.[1]

STEPS IN SYNAPTIC TRANSMISSION

The synapse is of such central importance to the functioning of the nervous system and to the action of psychoactive drugs that it will be useful to examine in more detail its structural features and its process of transferring information from the axon of one cell to the dendrites of another. Figure II.1 shows a schematic representation of a norepinephrine synapse (which can be considered a typical synapse). It may be seen that the axon terminal makes close approximation with the dendrite through a narrow space of about 200 Å. This space (the synaptic cleft) separates the presynaptic membrane (the axon and axon terminal) from the postsynaptic membrane of the dendrite. In the presynaptic terminal are found mitochrondria (the metabolic factories of the cell) and numerous small synaptic vesicles. These vesicles are approximately 300 to 600 Å in diameter and in the nervous system are almost universally found in the nerve terminals adjacent to the presynaptic membrane on the presynaptic side of the cleft. In fact, the presence of these synaptic vesicles is considered proof of the presence of a synapse. Transmitter chemical is stored in these vesicles before it is released. The postsynaptic membrane is similar to membranes found elsewhere in the nervous system.

This, then, is the general organization of the synapse. Structure alone, however, does not explain the sequence of events that

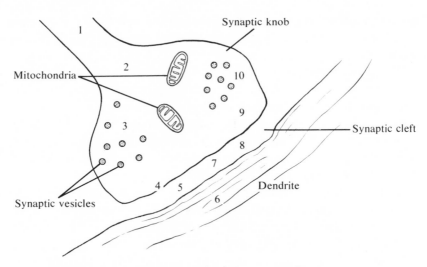

1. Conduction of the action potential down the presynaptic axon.
2. Arrival of the action potential at the nerve terminal.
3. Synthesis of NE (see Figure II.5) and storage of NE in the synaptic vesicles (this may occur before steps 1 and 2).
4. Release of NE from synaptic vesicles into the synaptic cleft upon the arrival of an action potential.
5. Diffusion of NE across the synaptic cleft.
6. Stimulation of the postsynaptic receptors by NE.
7. Release of NE from postsynaptic receptors back into the synaptic cleft.
8. Metabolism of some of the NE in the synaptic cleft by extracellular enzymes.
9. Uptake of some of the NE back into the presynaptic nerve terminal.
10. Uptake of NE in the presynaptic nerve terminal into the synaptic vesicles where it is protected from destruction by the enzyme MAO.

Figure II.1. Schematic diagram of a norepinephrine (NE) synapse within the central nervous system. The steps in the transmission of information across such a synapse are numbered in the diagram and listed below it.

occurs between the arrival of an action potential at the terminal of one axon and the alterations that are then produced in the postsynaptic membrane of the dendrite of the next neuron. Basically there are 10 steps to consider in the synaptic transmission process (numbered in Figure II.1). Steps 1 through 4 are presynaptic events involving the synthesis, storage, and release of neurotransmitter. Steps 5 through 8 involve the extracellular action of the transmitter; that is, diffusion, receptor activation, and metabolic destruction of transmitter. Steps 9 and 10 involve the reuptake of the chemical transmitter and result in the cessation of information transfer. Step 9 involves the special property of the presynaptic membrane selectively to take up transmitter back into the presynaptic nerve terminal, thus removing it from the synaptic cleft. Finally, step 10 is the active reuptake of the transmitter that is in intracellular fluid inside the nerve terminal back into the synaptic vesicles where the transmitter is protected from intracellular enzymes that might otherwise destroy it.

CRITERIA FOR A TRANSMITTER SUBSTANCE

Since the evidence for chemical transmission between neurons is virtually conclusive and since the steps in synaptic transmission have been identified, a vigorous search for specific transmitter substances in the central nervous system is currently in progress. A number of criteria must be satisfied in order to prove conclusively that a chemical is in fact an excitatory or inhibitory transmitter at a given synapse (Table II.1).

Table II.1. Criteria for a Chemical Neurotransmitter

1. The proposed compound must be contained within the presynaptic nerve terminal.
2. The proposed compound must be released from nerve endings on stimulation of the nerve.
3. Injection of the proposed neurotransmitter must mimic the synaptic action that occurs after the normal transmitter is released.
4. There must be some mechanism (enzymatic or otherwise) by which transmitter action can be terminated and that fits the time course of transmitter action.
5. Drugs that interfere with the actions of the proposed transmitter must exert an identical action upon the effects of nerve stimulation.

Common sense would dictate that one criterion would be that the transmitter chemical must be contained within the presynaptic terminal or that at least an immediate precursor (a substance that eventually becomes the transmitter) must be present. Strangely enough, for some of the substances discussed below, even this most essential criterion has not been satisfied conclusively. By similar reasoning, it would seem that this transmitter substance in the presynaptic terminal must be released from the synaptic nerve ending in response to the arrival of an action potential. In the peripheral nervous system, this second criterion is relatively easily satisfied, but in the central nervous system it is more difficult, since it is almost impossible to stimulate one axon selectively and to collect any substance that is released from the terminals of that axon. The third criterion is that the injection of a suspected synaptic transmitter must exert an effect on the postsynaptic membrane identical to the effect that follows the release of the normal transmitter. The same technical difficulties hinder the satisfaction of both the second and third criteria. The fourth criterion is that there must be some mechanism (enzymatic or otherwise) by which the action of the transmitter can be terminated and that fits the time course of action of the transmitter substance. This criterion has been more easily satisfied, although there is still difficulty in pinpointing precisely the exact mechanisms involved. The fifth criterion is that drugs that are known to alter the synthesis, release, action, or degradation of a supposed transmitter substance must exert an identical action at the synapse in question.

To date, there are few sites in the brain where any suspected transmitter substance has been shown to meet all these criteria. It is not surprising, however, that more advances have not been made in this area since the technical difficulties of the isolation and study of single synapses in the brain are enormous. In the peripheral nerves, it is often relatively easy to isolate particular types of synapses, which may then be accurately identified.

SPECIFIC TRANSMITTER SUBSTANCES

In this section, we will discuss specific transmitter substances: acetylcholine, norepinephrine and dopamine, serotonin, and excitatory and inhibitory amino acids.

Acetylcholine

Acetylcholine was first identified as a transmitter chemical in the peripheral nervous system. We now know that it is present in large amounts in brain tissue. Thus, it is not too surprising that scientists have interpreted this to mean that acetylcholine is also a

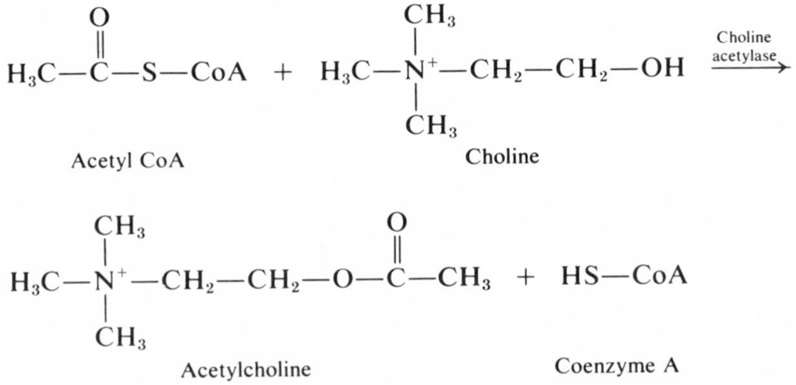

Figure II.2. Chemical reactions in the brain responsible for synthesis of acetylcholine. The acetylcholine is synthesized from acetyl CoA and choline.

transmitter chemical in the brain, so we shall discuss the evidence for and against the role of acetylcholine as a transmitter in the central nervous system.

The chemical reactions that take place in the nerve terminal and lead to the synthesis of acetylcholine are illustrated in Figure II.2, and the dynamics of the acetylcholine nerve terminal are portrayed in Figure II.3. Following synthesis, acetylcholine is thought to be stored inside the nerve terminal within synaptic vesicles until it is released into the synaptic cleft upon arrival of an action potential from the axon. The acetylcholine then diffuses across the cleft and attaches itself to receptors on the dendrite of the next neuron, which results in the transmission of information between the two neurons. This attachment is important to the pharmacologist since some psychoactive drugs may either mimic the action of acetylcholine at

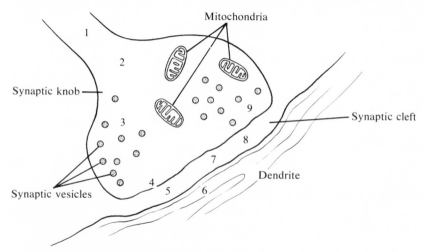

1. Conduction of the action potential down the presynaptic axon.
2. Arrival of the action potential at the nerve terminal.
3. Synthesis of ACh (see Figure II.2) and storage of ACh in the synaptic vesicles (this may occur before steps 1 and 2).
4. Release of ACh from synaptic vesicles into the synaptic cleft upon the arrival of an action potential.
5. Diffusion of ACh across the synaptic cleft.
6. Stimulation of the postsynaptic receptors by ACh.
7. Release of ACh from postsynaptic receptors back into the synaptic cleft.
8. Metabolism of ACh in the synaptic cleft by the enzyme AChE (see Figure II.4).
9. Uptake of choline produced by metabolism of ACh into the presynaptic nerve terminal for the resynthesis of ACh.

Figure II.3. Schematic diagram of an acetylcholine (ACh) synapse. The steps in transmission of information across such a synapse are numbered in the diagram and listed below it.

the dendritic receptor or else block access of the transmitter to the receptor. Drugs that mimic the action of acetylcholine at the receptor include compounds such as nicotine and muscarine, both of which may alter behavior. Agents thought to block access of acetylcholine to the receptors include atropine and scopolamine.

Once acetylcholine has exerted its effect on the postsynaptic dendritic membrane, its action must somehow be terminated. Acetylcholine is destroyed by an enzyme, acetylcholine esterase (AChE). The process is illustrated in Figure II.4. The reaction that destroys acetylcholine is important to the pharmacologist because many drugs (referred to as AChE inhibitors) will inhibit the destructive enzyme. Such drugs include physostigmine, malathion, parathion, sarin, and soman, all of which may induce nightmares, confusion, hallucinations, feelings of agitation, confusion, and a slowing of intellectual and motor functions.

At present, the localization of acetylcholine in the brain is poorly delineated. Through indirect evidence it is thought that the highest concentrations of acetylcholine are in the caudate nucleus, certain brainstem nuclei, and the cerebral cortex. Little else is known about the role of acetylcholine in brain function. It is not yet even clear whether acetylcholine is an excitatory transmitter (producing EPSPs) or an inhibitory transmitter (producing IPSPs). It is entirely possible that it may be both excitatory and inhibitory, depending upon the reaction of the postsynaptic membrane to the chemical, because if one takes a microelectrode (a glass pipette with a tip that has a diameter of between 1 and 10 microns) and places acetylcholine directly onto individual cells within the brain, one finds that the acetylcholine increases the discharge of some neurons and inhibits the discharge of others.

Norepinephrine and Dopamine

The term *catecholamine* refers to a group of chemically related compounds, the most important of which are epinephrine, norepinephrine, and dopamine. In the peripheral nervous system, epinephrine is a neurotransmitter important in the maintenance of such major body functions as blood pressure and heart rate. Epinephrine is not commonly found in the brain. During the last 10 years, a large body of evidence has accumulated to demonstrate that norepinephrine and dopamine are the catecholamine neurotransmitters in the brain. This evidence appears to be much more substantial than

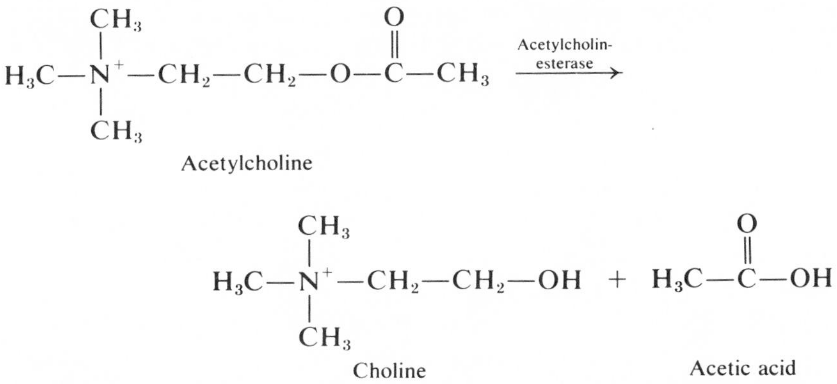

$$CH_3 \quad\quad\quad O$$
$$| \quad\quad\quad\quad\quad ||$$
$$H_3C-N^+-CH_2-CH_2-O-C-CH_3 \xrightarrow{\text{Acetylcholin-esterase}}$$
$$|$$
$$CH_3$$

Acetylcholine

$$CH_3 \quad\quad\quad\quad\quad\quad\quad O$$
$$| \quad\quad\quad\quad\quad\quad\quad\quad ||$$
$$H_3C-N^+-CH_2-CH_2-OH \;+\; H_3C-C-OH$$
$$|$$
$$CH_3$$

Choline   Acetic acid

Figure II.4. Destruction of acetylcholine (ACh) by the enzyme acetyl-cholinesterase (AChE).

that on acetylcholine, primarily because researchers can locate precisely the catecholamines in the brain. It has also become clear that many drugs that profoundly affect brain function and behavior exert their effects by altering the synaptic action of norepinephrine and dopamine in the brain. In many instances, the effects of new drugs on behavior have been predicted because of knowledge of their effects on the actions of the catecholamine neurotransmitters.

Dopamine and norepinephrine are manufactured within catecholamine neurons by the steps shown in Figure II.5. This synthesis was first proposed in 1939 and has now been confirmed, and the enzymes involved in each step have been identified and intensively studied. We shall not discuss the details of this scheme except to mention the step involving the enzyme tyrosine hydroxylase as a catalyst. Inhibition of this enzyme by drugs such as α-methyl-p-tyrosine results in a reduction in brain catecholamines and induces sedation, apparently secondary to the enzyme's inhibition of NE synthesis, which would indicate that the levels and functioning of neurotransmitters within the brain underlie behavior. By a similar reasoning, one might assume that drugs that alter behavior probably produce their effects secondary to alterations in chemical transmission between neurons. In Parkinson's disease, the dopamine normally present in a part of the brain called the caudate nucleus is reduced in amount. Administration of dopamine into the body is of little therapeutic use since it does not cross the blood-brain barrier. However, the administration of Dopa (the precursor to dopamine) does increase the dopamine levels in the caudate nucleus. What appears to happen is that Dopa is capable of crossing the blood-brain barrier and

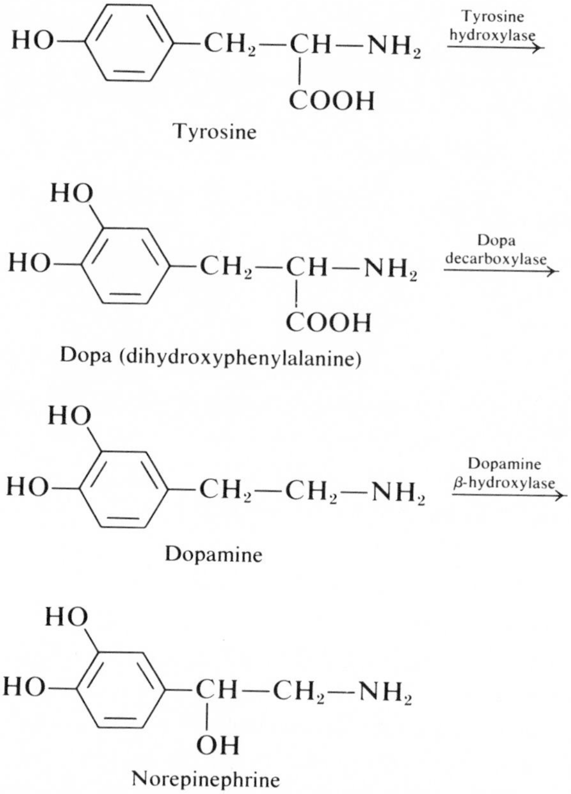

Figure II.5. Synthesis of norepinephrine (NE) from tyrosine. Note the intermediate compounds formed in this reaction; namely, Dopa and dopamine.

is converted to dopamine in the brain. This is an example of how knowledge of the chemical synthesis of a transmitter may be used to clinical benefit.

METABOLIC FATE

A transmitter must be synthesized, released, exert a postsynaptic effect, and then be inactivated. Inactivation can occur by either or both of two processes: enzymatic destruction, and reuptake of the transmitter from the synaptic cleft back into the presynaptic nerve terminal. Catecholamines are inactivated by the enzymes monoamine oxidase (MAO) and catechol o-methyltransferase (COMT) (Figure II.6). Because these enzymatic inactivations appear to be less important in the termination of dopamine or norepinephrine neurotransmission than is the destruction of acetylcholine by AChE, it is unlikely that the postsynaptic effects of dopamine or norepinephrine are terminated to any significant extent by enzymes. The actions of these

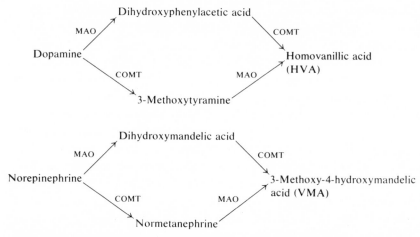

Figure II.6. Destruction of dopamine and norepinephrine. The inactivating enzymes are monoamine oxidase (MAO) and catechol o-methyltransferase (COMT).

transmitters are terminated primarily by an active process of their reuptake across the presynaptic nerve membrane back into the presynaptic nerve ending. Norepinephrine or dopamine taken up in this way is then stored again in the synaptic vesicles, to be reused.

The principle of reuptake into the nerve terminal and then into the storage vesicles is of crucial importance, since there are drugs that may block either the active uptake process into the nerve terminal (thus potentiating the synaptic action of the transmitter) or the uptake of the transmitter from the intracellular fluid in the nerve terminal back into the synaptic vesicles. Reserpine is an example of a drug that blocks this uptake into the vesicle; cocaine is a representative of a class of drugs that block reuptake from the synaptic cleft into the nerve terminal. (As stated in chapters 5 and 7, reserpine and cocaine have nearly opposite effects on the body and the brain.)

THE CATECHOLAMINE SYNAPSE

The dynamics of dopamine and norepinephrine are only slightly different from those of other CNS transmitters. A norepinephrine synapse is illustrated in Figure II.1. It is similar to the acetylcholine terminal presented in Figure II.3—that is, the presynaptic nerve terminal contains mitochondria and small vesicles containing stored transmitter. Also, like the acetylcholine terminal, the presynaptic nerve terminal is separated from the postsynaptic dendritic membrane by a distance of approximately 200 Å. The dopamine and norepinephrine terminals, however, contain entirely different chemical products. The amino acid tyrosine (obtained from food) is taken into the presynaptic terminal, where it is transformed to Dopa, dopamine, and, in some terminals, norepinephrine (NE).

In those terminals in which dopamine is not transformed into NE, the dopamine itself serves as the transmitter substance. The transmitter is stored in the synaptic vessels until released. Upon arrival of an action potential at the nerve terminal, the norepinephrine (or dopamine) is released from the vesicles (which cluster close to the cleft) into the synaptic cleft. The transmitter then diffuses across the cleft, reacting with the postsynaptic membrane to transfer information from one neuron to another. The transmission process is terminated by the uptake of NE (or dopamine) back into the nerve terminal, where it is either metabolized by the intracellular enzyme MAO or else taken up into and stored by the vesicles until it is released again.

At present, our knowledge of the functional role of norepinephrine in the brain is limited, in part, by a lack of understanding about which specific behavioral responses are associated with NE neurons. There is circumstantial evidence that the activity of neurons containing norepinephrine is associated with arousal reactions and with mood. This is illustrated by the fact that emotionally intense experiences (such as anxiety, fright, anger, and expectation) are accompanied by release of epinephrine in the peripheral nervous system. It is likely that norepinephrine neurons in the brain act similarly and are a representation of this "sympathetic" nervous system in the rest of the body. This hypothesis was postulated in the early 1950s when reserpine was introduced as a tranquilizing agent and the drug's sedative action was correlated with a depletion of norepinephrine in the brain. Since then, many of the inferences about the functions of NE and dopamine have been drawn from recent work on the location of these substances in the brain.

LOCALIZATION IN BRAIN

In recent years, much has been learned about the precise localization of dopamine and norepinephrine neurons and synapses within the brain. The cell somas and dendrites are situated in one area of the brain and the axons travel to other sites in the brain, where they synapse with the dendrites of other cells. In discussing the localization of dopamine and norepinephrine in the brain, we have to consider both the sites of the cell bodies (somas) and the sites to which their axons project. Figure II.7 is a schematic diagram of the

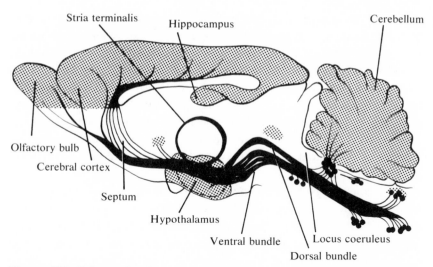

Figure II.7. Schematic diagram of distribution of NE in rat brain. This illustrates the distribution of the main ascending pathways that contain norepinephrine as the synaptic transmitter. The shaded areas indicate the major nerve-terminal areas. [Modified from U. Ungerstedt, "Adipsia and Aphagia After 6-hydroxydopamine Induced Degeneration of the Nigro-striatal Dopamine System," *Acta Physiologica Scandinavica,* supplement 367 (1971): fig. 6, p. 110.]

distribution of norepinephrine in the brain. It appears that most norepinephrine cell bodies are situated in the brainstem and that these cell bodies send axons to certain brain structures. Other cell bodies send axons from the brainstem down to the spinal cord. Since the lower brain and the brainstem appear to be essential to the display of basic instinctual behavior in hunger, thirst, emotion, and sex, norepinephrine may be a neurotransmitter important in the regulation of these functions. More will be said about the physiology and pharmacology of the brainstem in Appendix III.

Dopamine cell bodies are primarily situated in the substantia nigra. These cells send axons to a group of structures called the *basal ganglia.* The dopamine neurons play an important role in movement, and loss of dopamine is associated with the disease called Parkinsonism. Thus, dopamine neurons appear to be clearly distinguishable from norepinephrine neurons.

DRUG EFFECTS ON NE NERVE TERMINALS

Figure II.1 illustrates the general organization of a nerve terminal, with its processes of synthesis, storage, release, metabolism, and reuptake of transmitter, using a norepinephrine terminal as an example. There are many drugs that are capable of inhibiting each of these processes in norepinephrine neurotransmission. Some drugs are capable of interfering with the synthesis of NE—for example, α-methyl-p-tyrosine and α-methyldopa. The latter compound is used clinically as an antihypertensive (the drug lowers blood pressure). Some drugs are capable of blocking the reuptake of norepinephrine from the synaptic cleft back into the nerve terminal, thus increasing the action of NE at the synapse. Such compounds include cocaine and a series of drugs that elevate mood and reverse depression (the tricyclic antidepressants).

Some drugs are capable of blocking the movement of norepinephrine from the intracellular fluid in the presynaptic nerve terminal into the storage granule (synaptic vesicle) where the transmitter is stored and protected from the enzyme MAO. An example of such a drug is reserpine. As a result of this blockage, NE may be metabolized by MAO and the nervous system depleted of the transmitter, with the result being sedation and emotional depression. Some drugs are capable of blocking the enzyme MAO, thereby increasing the NE concentration in the nerve terminal. Tranylcypromine (Parnate) is one such MAO inhibitor; this action appears to account for the ability of the drug to elevate mood and reverse depression, effects similar to those produced by cocaine. Some compounds (ephedrine, for example) are capable of stimulating the postsynaptic norepinephrine receptor; others (phenoxybenzamine, for example) are capable of blocking the receptor. Some drugs, such as amphetamine, are capable of inducing the release of norepinephrine from the nerve terminal.

Serotonin

Serotonin (also called 5-hydroxytryptamine or 5-HT), like acetylcholine, norepinephrine, and dopamine, is believed to be a neurotransmitter in the brain. When 5-HT was first found within the brain, the theory arose that mental illness might be due to biochemical abnormalities within the 5-HT system. Current thought holds that this may be partly true, but mental illness is not so simply explained and other neurotransmitters are undoubtedly involved. Reserpine, for example, induces profound mental depression, apparently by depleting both norepinephrine and 5-HT.

More recently, several hallucinogenic compounds (LSD, for example) have been found to resemble 5-HT structurally, and the hypothesis has been advanced that at least some drug-induced hallucinations are due to alterations in the functioning of 5-HT neurons.

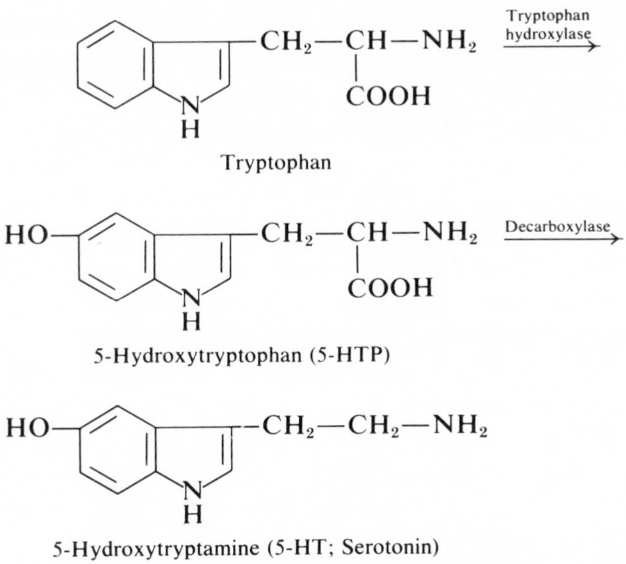

Figure II.8. Synthesis of 5-hydroxytryptamine (serotonin) from tryptophan.

In the brain, significant amounts of 5-HT are found in the upper brainstem. In the body, large amounts of 5-HT are found in the intestinal tract. The biosynthesis of 5-HT is illustrated in Figure II.8. The drug p-chlorophenylalanine (PCPA) inhibits the enzyme tryptophan hydroxylase, resulting in the depletion of 5-HT, with the concomitant induction of insomnia. An animal given PCPA will not sleep for several days, an effect that has generated much speculation on the role of 5-HT in sleep.

Like norepinephrine and dopamine, 5-HT is destroyed by the enzyme MAO. Metabolism of 5-HT results in formation of 5-hydroxyindoleacetic acid (5-HIAA). Several hypotheses about a link between levels of 5-HT and mental illness (especially schizophrenia) have followed observations of altered levels of 5-HIAA in the urine of mentally ill patients. In the brain, 5-HT appears to be a neurotransmitter involved in the regulation of body temperature, sensory perception, and sleep. Its other functions are less clear.

Excitatory and Inhibitory Amino Acids

Since specific roles of excitatory and inhibitory amino acids in behavioral function are poorly delineated, these compounds will be only briefly discussed. They must be mentioned, however, because extensive research within the last few years indicates that certain amino acids may play important roles in the brain as neurotransmitter

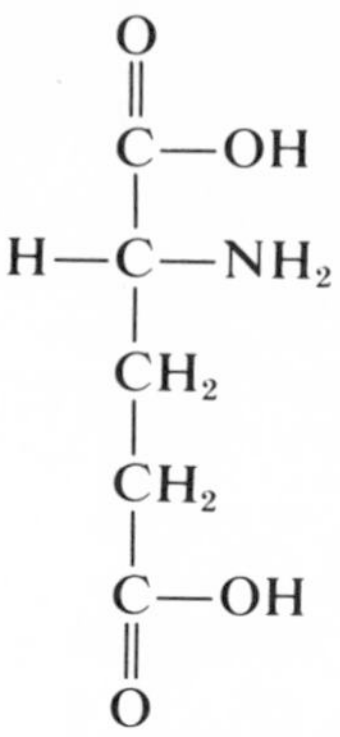

Glutamic acid

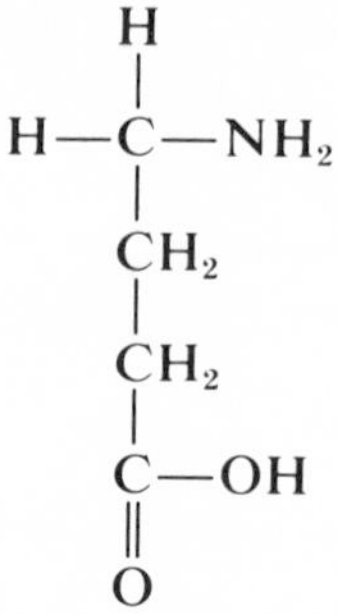

γ-Aminobutyric acid (Gaba)

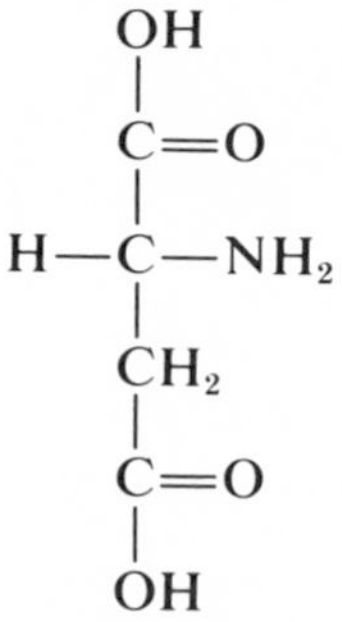

Aspartic acid

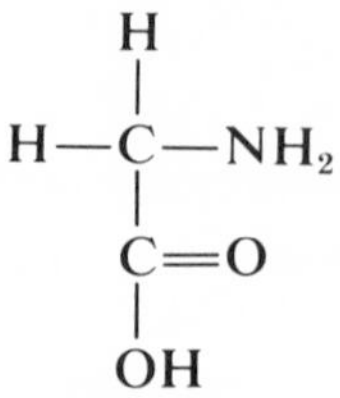

Glycine

Figure II.9. Structures of four possible chemical neurotransmitters within CNS.

substances. The brain contains high concentrations of aspartic acid, γ-aminobutyric acid (Gaba), and glutamic acid, and the spinal cord contains high concentrations of glycine. The structures of these four compounds are presented in Figure II.9.

Aspartic acid and glutamic acid appear to be universally excitatory; that is, their application to virtually any brain cell results in increased activity of that cell. Gaba and the glycine appear to be universally inhibitory. Interference with the activity of Gaba or glycine synapses usually leads to convulsions. However, the precise role of these excitatory and inhibitory amino acids in the brain is still not clear. They appear to regulate brain excitability and may have important roles in behavior.

OTHER PUTATIVE NEUROTRANSMITTER SUBSTANCES

To date, the major thrust of investigations of possible neurotransmitter substances in the brain has centered upon acetylcholine, norepinephrine, dopamine, serotinin, and the amino acids. Other substances have also been studied as possible neurotransmitters, among them histamine, the exact function of which is still obscure. It is well known, however, that the administration of antihistamines (drugs that block the action of histamine) induces sedation. Whether this sedation is due to an action of these drugs on histamine synapses is as yet unclear. Other proposed neurotransmitters include the prostaglandins, ergothioneine, substance P, and many others. There is as yet, however, insufficient evidence to consider these compounds seriously as neurotransmitters involved in behavior and as possible sites of action of psychoactive drugs.

(This brief review of neurotransmitters has been necessarily introductory. For a more complete discussion of drug action on central synapses, see the monograph by Cooper, Bloom, and Roth.[2])

NOTES

1. G. B. Koelle, "Neurohumoral Transmission and the Autonomic Nervous System," in *The Pharmacological Basis of Therapeutics,* 5th ed. L. S. Goodman and A. Gilman, eds. (New York: Macmillan, 1975), pp. 410–12.

2. J. R. Cooper, F. E. Bloom, and R. H. Roth, *The Biochemical Basis of Neuropharmacology,* 2d ed. (New York: Oxford University Press, 1974).

Basic Anatomy of the Nervous System

In appendixes I and II, we discussed the neuron as the fundamental unit of the nervous system and the synapse and chemical neurotransmitters as the means of communication between individual neurons. In this appendix, we will go one step further and discuss the neurons as functional units within specific areas of the brain. It seems logical that we would have a better understanding of the actions of psychoactive drugs after we make an introductory examination of the functions of the nervous system that underlie behavior.

Since the brain is perhaps the most complex of all biological structures, discussion of its anatomy and function is difficult. Still, a number of introductory and straightforward principles can be described that may lead to a relatively uncomplicated outline of the anatomy and physiology of the brain and help explain why different drugs acting at different synapses exert different effects on brain function and on behavior.

INTRODUCTORY TERMINOLOGY

For ease in teaching and in understanding, the nervous system is divided into two major functional systems: the *central nervous system (CNS)* and the *peripheral nervous system*. The central nervous system consists of all the neurons that are situated inside the skull and the spine. The peripheral nervous system consists of all the

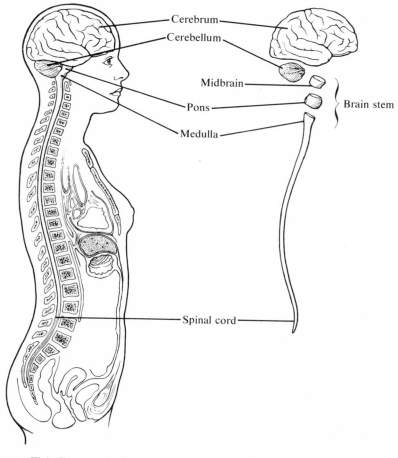

Figure III.1. The central nervous system. The situation of the brain and spinal cord within the body *(left)* and the principal components of the central nervous system *(right)*.

neurons outside the skull and spine. In turn, the CNS may be sub-divided into two major parts: the brain and the spinal cord. The brain is a collection of some 13 billion neurons, with their dendrites and axons, entirely contained within the skull (Figure III.1). The lower part of the brain, which is attached to the upper part of the spinal cord, is referred to as the *brainstem*. The brainstem is situated en-tirely within the skull. All impulses transmitted (in both directions) between the spinal cord and the brain must of necessity be transmit-ted through the brainstem, which is also important in the regulation of vital body functions and is a site of action of many psychoactive drugs.

If we divide the brain into its component parts (Figure III.1), we see that the top or front end of the CNS (the *cerebrum*) is consid-erably larger than the brainstem and the spinal cord. As the upper part of the spinal cord enlarges, it separates into three distinct yet completely interconnected segments, referred to as the *medulla,* the *pons* (or bridge) and the *midbrain*. Collectively, the brainstem comprises these three segments. The area immediately above the brainstem is referred to as the *diencephalon* and includes the hypothalamus, the pituitary gland, the fiber tracts from the eyes (op-tic tracts), the thalamus, and the region below the thalamus referred to as the subthalamus. Finally, almost completely covering the brainstem and diencephalon are the two *cerebral hemispheres,* the left and the right.

Although this is not a complete outline of all brain structures (several structures have been omitted), this should suffice as an intro-duction to the concept that the brain is not a homogeneous structure but may be subdivided anatomically into many functional units.

THE SPINAL CORD

The spinal cord, in general, handles two types of activities: the spinal reflexes and the channeling of information between the periphery and the brain. If you step on a tack or touch a hot stove, you will immediately withdraw the affected limb. This unconscious reflex withdrawal in response to heat or pain is carried out over an arrangement of neurons called a *reflex arc* set up through the spinal cord. When you step on a tack, sensory receptors are stimulated. These receptors are specialized dendrites of neurons whose sole func-tion is to sense the external environment. In contrast to the typical neuron discussed in Appendix I, the dendrite of this sensory receptor is activated by heat, cold, pain, touch, or pressure rather than by chemically induced synaptic EPSPs. This specialized neuron sends information to the spinal cord, where (through a synapse) a motor neuron is excited (by an EPSP). Excitation of the motor neuron is translated into action potentials that travel to the muscles, which then contract and cause the withdrawal from the painful stimulus.

The motor neurons in the spinal cord are also influenced by information from the brain. For example, certain areas of the brain when stimulated will increase the activity of the motor neurons. Many drugs that cause behavioral sedation decrease the flow of information from the brain to the spinal cord. Such drugs are frequently used as muscle relaxants because they decrease the spinal cord's control over muscle tone by indirectly decreasing the activity of the motor neurons. Other drugs can produce just the opposite effect. For example, some convulsant drugs, such as strychnine, block inhibitory controls over the activity of the motor neurons. Discharges from the motor neurons are increased and convulsions result.

THE BRAINSTEM

The brainstem lies inside the skull and connects the spinal cord with the diencephalon and the cerebrum. The major subdivisions of the brainstem are the *medulla, pons,* and *midbrain* (Figure III.1). Behind the midbrain is a large bulbous structure called the *cerebellum.*

Medulla

The medulla is the direct continuation of the spinal cord in the skull. All ascending and descending fiber tracts connecting the brain and the spinal cord pass through the medulla. Also, in the medulla are centers largely responsible for the control of respiration (breathing), peripheral vasoconstriction (blood pressure), heart rate, strength of contraction of the heart, functioning of the gastrointestinal tract, and control of sleeping and waking. The medulla also seems to play a fundamental role in behavioral alerting, attention, or arousal. Some depressant drugs (such as the opiates and the barbiturates) depress these centers in the brainstem, and death from an overdose of such drugs may occur as a result of the depression of the centers. Other agents that are clinically used for the treatment of high blood pressure seem to exert at least part of their hypotensive effect by depressing the centers in the medulla that control vascular tone. Drugs that affect the state of arousal of an animal or affect sleeping or wakefulness seem to act in the medulla and in the rest of the brainstem.

All drug actions on the brainstem, however, are not depressant in nature. Some drugs exert both stimulant and depressant effects, depending on the specific area. Morphine, for example, depresses respiratory centers in the medulla, but it also stimulates an area in the medulla called the chemoreceptor trigger zone. Stimulation of this zone may result in vomiting.

The central core of the medulla is a complex network of cell bodies (somas) and fibers (axons) that extends from the medulla up the brainstem almost to the level of the thalamus and is called the *reticular formation*. One portion of this reticular formation is referred to as the *ascending reticular activating system (ARAS)*. In 1949, it was demonstrated that electrical stimulation of the ARAS resulted in a transition in the brain-wave activity (the electroencephalogram, or EEG) from that characteristic of sleep to that characteristic of wakefulness. Destruction of the ARAS tended to yield an EEG pattern that is usually associated with drowsiness or sleep. Thus, it would seem, by association, that the ARAS is involved in the control of sleeping and waking (and also behavioral alerting). It was subsequently demonstrated in the mid-1950s that drugs that produce depression (the barbiturates and ether, for example) inhibit activity in the ARAS.

The ARAS is stimulated normally by inputs passing through the brainstem en route from the body to the brain. The resulting activation of the cortex by the ARAS may alert the brain to be ready to receive information. If the ARAS could not be activated by incoming information, the animal would be unaware of its surroundings and would most likely be asleep or not receptive. Barbiturates, for example (see Chapter 3), depress the ARAS so that it is not excited by incoming information and stimuli do not arouse the animal (that is, the animal is asleep or anesthetized).

Drugs that stimulate the ARAS would be expected to arouse the animal and most probably increase behavioral activity. Amphetamine, one such drug, is thought to stimulate behavior by increasing the activity of norepinephrine synapses in the ARAS.

More recently, evidence has been presented that antipsychotic drugs such as chlorpromazine (Chapter 7) may exert their actions by decreasing input into the ARAS and that psychedelic compounds such as LSD (Chapter 8) may exert their actions of intensifying alertness and causing hallucinations by increasing input into the ARAS.

Pons

The pons (or bridge) is the part of the brainstem above the medulla and below the midbrain. The pons contains ascending and descending fiber tracts (axons) connecting the brain, the spinal cord, and the cerebellum and also contains a few structures that control sensory and motor functions to and from the face and head. To date, specific pharmacological actions on the pons have not been clearly delineated.

Midbrain

Above the pons is the midbrain. Toward the cerebrum, the midbrain merges with the thalamus, hypothalamus, and a large number of subthalamic structures. The outstanding features of the midbrain are the relay structures that control vision and hearing. Other structures in the midbrain control eye movement and muscle coordination. On the posterior of the midbrain are two structures called the inferior colliculus and the superior colliculus, which are important relay points in the auditory and visual systems and are thought to be possible sites of action of certain psychedelic drugs that induce auditory or visual hallucinations. The ARAS extends forward from the medulla up through the midbrain.

Cerebellum

The cerebellum is a large, highly convoluted structure situated immediately behind the brainstem and connected to it by three large pairs of fiber tracts. The exact functions of the cerebellum are still being studied, but it is quite widely agreed that the cerebellum is necessary for the proper integration of movement. Some drugs exert noticeable effects on cerebellar activity. Drunkenness, characterized by loss of coordination, staggering, loss of balance, and other deficits, appears to be largely due to an alcohol-induced depression of the cerebellum.

THE DIENCEPHALON

The diencephalon is a portion of the brain situated above the brainstem, below the cerebral cortex, and buried between the right and left cerebral hemispheres. The diencephalon may be further subdivided into several areas, three of which will be discussed: the thalamus, the hypothalamus, and the subthalamus.

Thalamus

The thalamus is the largest structure of the diencephalon and is actually a group of many smaller structures. Physiologically, the thalamus is often referred to as a way station, where incoming sensory pathways traveling up the spinal cord and through the brainstem synapse before passing into various areas of the cerebral cortex. Thus, the thalamus may be thought of as one of the prime relay stations of the brain.

Various subdivisions of the thalamus receive projections from specific sensory organs and, in turn, the neurons in these subdivisions relay information to specific areas of cerebral cortex. Inputs from vision, hearing, touch, pressure, position, pain, and so on feed into specific regions of the thalamus before being relayed to the areas of the cerebral cortex specifically associated with the senses. Other less well-defined areas of the thalamus are referred to as association areas. These areas do not receive sensory information directly but somehow integrate incoming information and relay it to the so-called association areas of the cerebral cortex. There are certain other areas of the thalamus that do not project directly to the cerebral cortex but connect the ARAS and the rest of the reticular formation with other thalamic regions, with the hypothalamus, and with the limbic system. These areas appear to form what is called the diffuse thalamic projection system, which has been implicated as a site of action of several psychoactive drugs. Electrical stimulation of the diffuse thalamic projection system yields behavioral alerting and EEG arousal reactions similar to those that follow stimulation of the ARAS. This diffuse thalamic projection system may therefore be an extension of the ARAS.

Subthalamus

The subthalamus is a small area underneath the thalamus and above the midbrain containing a variety of small structures that, in general, constitute one of our motor systems, the extrapyramidal system. In birds and lower mammals, this system is a motor system; it appears to be more important in the control of behavior and movements, it was found that the neurotransmitter dopamine was reduced however, the subthalamus is quite important. In patients with Parkinson's disease, a disorder characterized by exaggerated motor movements, it was found that the neurotransmitter dopamine was reduced in amount in the terminals of axons that originated from cell bodies in the substantia nigra (one of the subthalamic structures). Thus, in humans, as well as in lower mammals and birds, the subthalamic structures, together with the cerebellum, seem to be important in the control and coordination of motor activity.

Hypothalamus

The hypothalamus consists of a collection of structures in the lower portion of the brain near the junction of the midbrain and the thalamus. The hypothalamus has important centers for the control of such vegetative functions as eating, drinking, sleeping, the regulation of body temperature, sexual behavior, and water balance. (More intensive discussions of the functional anatomy of the hypothalamus and limbic system may be found in textbooks of physiological psychology listed in the bibliography. The structures are mentioned here, albeit briefly, because their functions are altered by many psychoactive drugs.) In addition, activity of the pituitary gland (Chapter 10) is under the close control of the hypothalamus. The hypothalamus also appears to be important in the modulation of emotion and behavior and is a site of action of many psychoactive drugs, either as a site of the drug's primary action or as a site responsible for side effects associated with the use of the drug. It is pertinent to mention the so-called reward centers in the hypothalamus, the self-stimulation centers, especially the posterior hypothalamus and other areas of the median forebrain bundle and the limbic system, which appear to contain norepinephrine neurons and to modulate what are referred to, in operant conditioning, as approach and avoidance behavior.

Limbic System

Closely associated with the hypothalamus is the limbic system, the major components of which are the amygdala, the hippocampus, the mammillary bodies, and a variety of other smaller structures. Recently, considerable attention has been drawn to the study of the effects of drugs on the hypothalamus and the limbic system. Since the limbic system and hypothalamus interact in the regulation of emotion and emotional expression, these structures are logical sites in which to study drugs that alter emotion or responses to emotional experiences. It is felt that some tranquilizers such as chlordiazepoxide (Librium) or diazepam (Valium) may depress limbic functions at doses below those that depress other functions of the brain. Such actions would result in "tranquilization" or "relief from anxiety" at doses lower than those that result in behavioral depression. The classical notion of the limbic system's being important in learning and memory have prompted investigations of this structure and the hypothalamus as sites of action of compounds that affect learning and memory. Atropine and scopolamine (Chapter 8) impair learning and memory and cause prominent alterations in electrical activity that may be recorded from the limbic system's structures. Certain structures of the limbic system have extremely low thresholds for seizure activity. It has been postulated (and in some cases demonstrated) that certain convulsant drugs act rather specifically upon structures of the limbic system.

The hypothalamus influences five categories of function: emotional behavior, eating and drinking behavior, sexual behavior, control of body functions (homeostasis), and control of the pituitary gland. It appears that the hypothalamus integrates emotional behavioral patterns. In the 1940s, W. R. Hess found that electrical stimulation of certain areas of the hypothalamus induced the sorts of responses usually encountered in expressions of rage. He suggested that these responses were part of the mechanisms in the brain and body that are normally involved in the mediation of the fight/flight/fright response. The fight/flight/fright reaction may be seen after the administration of such sympathomimetic drugs as amphetamine, which, for instance, increases activity apparently as a result of its action on the centers in the hypothalamus and the limbic system.

A satiety center is situated in one part of the hypothalamus, a feeding center in another. If the satiety center is destroyed, an animal will feed excessively and become obese; if the feeding and drinking centers are destroyed, an animal will neither eat nor drink. Amphetamine is a potent appetite suppressant and the drug has often been used clinically (although improperly) for this purpose. It is thought that amphetamine stimulates the neurons in the satiety center so that the animal stops eating because it feels full.

The hypothalamus is an important structure for both the neural and the humoral control of sexual behavior. If the front part of the hypothalamus is destroyed, an animal will not mate. Electrical stimulation of this part of the hypothalamus usually leads to increase in sexual behavior. Since most of the patterns observed during periods of sexual arousal are sympathetic in origin (for example, increased heart rate, increased blood pressure, and behavioral excitement), it is not surprising that this emotion would arise from a center in the brain that is involved in the control of the sympathetic nervous system. Much of the sex drive appears to be due to an action of neurons in the hypothalamus.

The hypothalamus is also important in the hormonal control of sex. Neurons in the hypothalamus produce and secrete substances called releasing factors, which travel to the nearby pituitary gland. There, they cause the production and secretion of hormones that act on the sex organs to cause sexual development, menstrual cycling, ovulation, and sperm formation. (The hypothalamus and pituitary gland are so active in the regulation of body hormones that Chapter 10 of this book was devoted entirely to this topic and to the action of drugs that affect fertility.)

We stated above that the hypothalamus is involved in a process of homeostasis. This merely means the hypothalamus is involved in the control of vital body functions such as temperature regulation and water balance. It appears that the hypothalamus contains discrete areas for the control of body temperature, one area being responsible for increasing body temperature and the other for decreasing it. If body temperature is increased, the anterior portion of the hypothalamus is activated and induces sweating and dilatation of cutaneous blood vessels, to aid the body in lowering its temperature. If body temperature (or skin temperature) drops, the posterior portion of the hypothalamus is activated and induces shivering and constriction of the cutaneous blood vessels in an effort to conserve heat.

Certain cells of the hypothalamus are osmoreceptors. This means that these cells are capable of responding to the osmolarity (salinity, saltiness) of the blood. These cells, by releasing antidiuretic hormone (ADH), control the ability of the body to retain fluids. If the osmolarity of the blood increases above normal, this is sensed by the osmoreceptor cells of the hypothalamus, ADH is released, and the kidneys respond by conserving rather than excreting body fluids. The hypothalamus is closely involved in the functioning of the pituitary gland, which may be regarded as the master gland of the body for, under the influence of the hypothalamus, it releases a number of hormones that control body function (see Chapter 10).

THE CEREBRAL CORTEX

In humans, the cerebral cortex makes up the largest portion of the brain. The cerebral cortex is separated into two distinct hemispheres, the left and the right. Numerous fiber tracts interconnect the two hemispheres both at a level above the thalamus and through multisynaptic pathways in the brainstem. In humans, since skull size is limited and the cerebral cortex has grown so large, the cortex is deeply convoluted and fissured. We will not discuss the functions of the cerebral cortex at length, but it is important to mention that, like the portions of the brain discussed above, the cerebral cortex is divided functionally—that is, it contains distinct centers for vision, hearing, speech, sensory perception, emotion, and so on.

The nervous system is extremely complex in structure and function and the cerebral cortex represents the ultimate development of this complexity. Volumes have been devoted to the structure and function of even small parts of the cerebral cortex, and only now are we becoming able to begin to understand something of the brain's precise functioning and interrelations. At present, little is known about the action of psychoactive drugs on the cerebral cortex. Undoubtedly, many psychoactive drugs will ultimately be found to affect the cerebral cortex, but our present knowledge of cortical function limits the precise delineation of such actions.

Appendix IV

Drug Transport

The absorption, distribution, metabolism, and excretion of drugs involve the passage of drugs across cell membranes. When we consider the passage of drugs out of the stomach and into the blood, we must take into account the fact that most drugs exist as a *mixture* of forms that are either water-soluble or fat-soluble. In the water-soluble form, the drug molecule exists in an electrically charged form called an ion and is therefore referred to as being ionized. The extent to which any given drug exists in either the water-soluble or the fat-soluble form depends on the drug itself and on the relative acidity of the fluid in which it is dissolved.

As we stated in Chapter 1, the body may be divided, theoretically, into several compartments, each of a different pH. The gastric juice is very acid (about pH 1.0), whereas the intestinal contents vary from about pH 2.0 to pH 6.6. Blood is slightly alkaline (pH 7.4), while the urine in the kidneys is acidic (usually between pH 4.5 and pH 7.0). The pH differences that therefore exist among blood, gastric juice, intestine, and kidney play a major role in determining whether a drug will be absorbed from an area of low pH to an area of higher pH or vice versa.

Most drugs are weak acids or bases and are present in solution in both un-ionized and ionized forms; the proportion of ionized drug to un-ionized drug depends upon the pK_a of the drug (the pH at which the drug is 50 percent ionized) and upon the acidity of the medium in which the drug is dissolved. The un-ionized portion is usually fat-soluble and can readily diffuse across cell membranes, but the ionized fraction is less able to penetrate most body membranes. The rate of equilibration of the un-ionized portion of a drug across the membrane is directly related to the drug's fat solubility since that is the limiting factor in determining passage through the membrane.

If a pH difference exists across the membrane (as for example, between stomach and blood), the fraction of ionized drug will be considerably greater on one side of the membrane than on the other. At equilibrium, the concentration of the un-ionized drug will be equal on both sides of the membrane; but the quantity of drug will be higher on the side where the degree of ionization is greater. This is illustrated in Figure IV.1, in which a weakly acidic drug is shown to exist in the gastric juice largely in the un-ionized (fat-soluble) form. Approximately 1,000 times as much of this particular drug exists in the un-ionized form as exists in the ionized form at this pH. In the blood, however, this weakly acidic drug exists largely in the ionized form, since it is now in an alkaline medium, so that approximately 1,000 times as much drug exists in the ionized form as exists in the un-ionized at this pH. Since un-ionized molecules are in equilibrium across the membrane, the concentrations of un-ionized drug will be the same in both compartments. However, as may be seen from Figure IV.1, there is a considerably larger quantity of drug in the blood than in the gastric juice since, in blood, the drug exists largely in the ionized form. Because these ionized drug molecules are unable to traverse the membrane back into the stomach, the drug is *absorbed* through this process of ion trapping. The ratio of un-ionized to ionized drug at each pH (and therefore in each compartment) can be calculated from the Henderson-Hasselbalch equation: pH = pK_a + log [base/acid].

Many drugs, however, are not weak acids but are weak *bases* (that is, they are slightly alkaline). In acidic compartments, such as

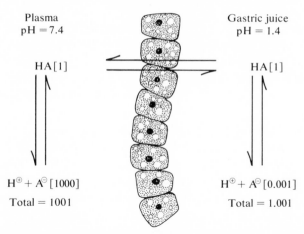

Figure IV.1. Compartmentalization of weakly acidic drug *(HA)* across cellular membrane separating stomach from blood. Note that in compartments of different pH, more or less of a drug will exist in an ionized or un-ionized form. Note also that only the un-ionized portion of the drug is in equilibrium across the membrane. [After E. Fingl and D. M. Woodbury, "General Principles," in *The Pharmacological Basis of Therapeutics,* 5th ed. L. S. Goodman and A. Gilman, eds. (New York: Macmillan, 1975), fig. 1-2, p. 4.]

the stomach, these weak bases are highly ionized and therefore do not pass through cell walls. In a basic (or alkaline) medium, however, such drugs are less ionized and exist largely in a fat-soluble form. A weak base is poorly absorbed from the stomach since it is highly ionized in gastric fluid and is ion-trapped in the stomach. In the

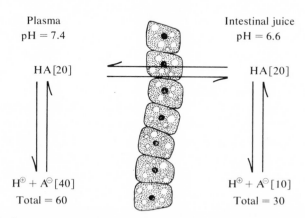

Figure IV.2. Compartmentalization of weak base drug *(HA)* across cellular membrane separating intestine from blood. Compare with Figure IV.1, which illustrates the distribution of a weak acid between the stomach and the blood. The difference of pH values in stomach and intestine allows for greatly different rates and degrees of absorption.

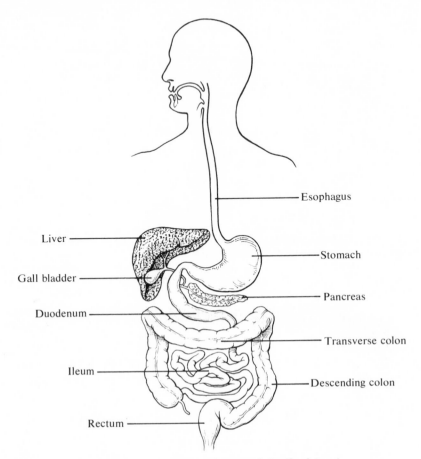

Figure IV.3. Schematic illustration of gastrointestinal tract.

intestine, however, the drug becomes less ionized and thus is better able to cross the membrane separating intestine from blood. This is illustrated in Figure IV.2, in which, in the intestine (pH 6.6), a weak base exists in both un-ionized and ionized forms. Slightly more of the drug is un-ionized. In the blood (pH 7.4), this same drug is more ionized than un-ionized (predictable from the Henderson-Hasselbalch equation). Thus, since only the un-ionized drug is in equilibrium across the membrane, there is a higher concentration of drug in the blood than in the intestine and the drug is absorbed. The absorption of weak bases from the intestine is much less complete than the absorption of weak acids from the stomach since there is a much smaller pH difference across the membrane. Therefore, absorption of drugs that are weak bases (compounds such as reserpine, codeine, morphine, or atropine) is much less efficient than absorption of weak acids and such drugs are often administered by injection.

The anatomy of the gastrointestinal tract is illustrated in Figure IV.3. Food (and drugs) must first pass through the stomach before they reach the intestine. Since weak acids are well absorbed from the stomach, large amounts frequently do not reach the intestine. Weak bases, however, are not absorbed from the stomach and must survive several hours exposure to stomach acids before they are passed into the intestine where they may be absorbed. This prolonged exposure to stomach acids tends to destroy many drugs and is another reason for the poor and incomplete absorption of weak bases that have been administered orally.

The Dose-Response Relationship

As we demonstrated in Chapter 1, there is little selectivity of distribution of drugs in the body. Psychoactive compounds are usually found fairly equally distributed to all tissues of the body (for example, there is usually as much drug in the liver or heart as there is in the brain). Thus, the selectivity of the compound (if any) is not dependent upon selective distribution of the drug but upon a selective distribution of receptors for the drug: the drug will act only where its receptors are situated. At different doses, the drug may interact with a variety of receptors. A drug, therefore, cannot be completely characterized by a single action since different effects will be observed at different doses. Few drugs exert only one effect.

One of the basic principles of pharmacology is that drug effects cannot be specifically delineated unless one considers the amount (or

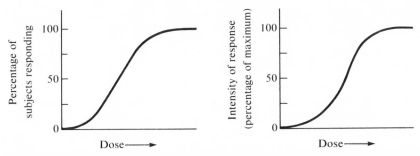

Figure V.1. Two types of dose-response curves. *Left,* the curve obtained by plotting the dose of drug against the percentage of subjects showing a given response at any given dose. *Right,* the dose of drug against the intensity of the response observed in any single individual at a given dose. The intensity of response is plotted as a percentage of the maximum obtainable response.

dose) of the drug. The relation between the dose of the drug and the intensity of a response is referred to as the *dose-response relation.* In Figure V.1 two types of dose-response curves are illustrated. In one case, the dose of the drug is plotted against the percentage of individuals exhibiting a characteristic effect. In the other example, the dose of the drug is plotted against the intensity or the magnitude of the response in a single individual. Both of these curves indicate that for each drug there is a dose low enough to produce no noticeable effect.

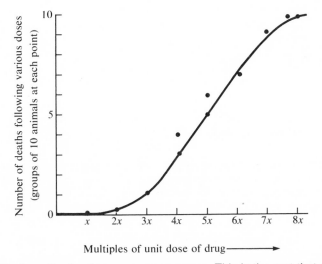

Figure V.2. A particular dose-response curve. This is the sort that would be obtained by plotting various doses of a drug against the deaths induced by progressive increases in dosage. Each point represents the number of deaths that occur in each group of 10 animals.

At the opposite extreme, there is a dose beyond which no greater response can be elicited. This dose-response relation is valid for only a single effect of the drug. Because every drug is capable of producing many effects, each drug will have a different dose-response curve for each observable effect that the drug induces. For example, for a sedative compound, a dose-response curve could be drawn for the amount of sedation induced. We could equally well draw a dose-response curve for the relation between the dose of drug and the number of animals put to sleep at each dose. Finally, we could draw a dose-response curve comparing the dose of the drug and the number of animals that died after the drug was administered (Figure V.2). For each comparison, however, the curve will be demonstrating three pertinent characteristics of the drug: its *potency* (from the position of the curve on the horizontal axis or the abscissa), its *slope* (the degree of intensification of response with a given increase in dose), and the dose required to produce the maximum effect. These three characteristics are illustrated in Figure V.3.

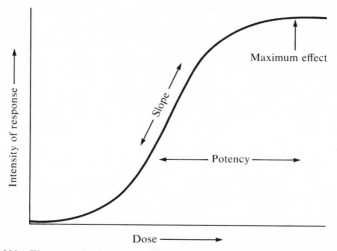

Figure V.3. Three principal components of dose-response curve: potency, slope, and maximum effect. [After E. Fingl and D. M. Woodbury, "General Principles," in *The Pharmacological Basis of Therapeutics,* 5th ed. L. S. Goodman and A. Gilman, eds. (New York: Macmillan, 1975), fig. 1–6, p. 25.]

POTENCY

The situation of the dose-response curve along the dose axis is an expression of the potency of the drug. We have all heard the statement that one drug is more potent than another, but what does this mean? Potency would obviously be influenced by the factors already discussed in this book—that is, absorption, distribution, metabolism, and excretion. For example, if two drugs are studied for their sedative effects but only one passes the blood-brain barrier, that drug would be the more potent. If both drugs were capable of producing sedation but one was capable of exerting this action at half the dose level of the other, the first drug would be considered as the more potent drug.

Potency, however, is a relatively unimportant characteristic of a drug, since it makes little difference whether the effective dose of a drug is 0.1 g or 10 g as long as the drug is administered in an appropriate dose and undue toxicity is not observed at that dose (a factor called *safety,* to be discussed below). Thus, there is little justification for the concept that the more potent the drug, the better it is. High potency, in fact, may be more of a disadvantage than an advantage, since an extremely potent drug may also be much more toxic (or dangerous) and therefore require much more careful handling.

SLOPE

Slope refers to the more or less linear, central portion of the dose-response curve. A steep dose-response curve (for a CNS depressant) implies that there is a smaller difference between the dose that produces death and the dose that causes mild sedation than would be observed with a depressant that had a lower slope. The steeper the slope, the smaller the increase in dose required to go from a minimal response to a maximal effect. The slope of the dose-response curve is one of the variables that must be considered in determining the relative safety of a drug.

MAXIMUM EFFECT

The peak of the dose-response curve indicates the maximum effect produced by a drug. Not all stimulant drugs, for example, are capable of exerting the same level of CNS stimulation. Caffeine, even in massive doses, is incapable of exerting the same intensity of CNS stimulation that is induced by amphetamine. Thus, maximum effect of a drug is an inherent property of a drug. Some drugs may be used to the point of maximum effect. However, with most pharmacological agents, undesired side effects limit the upper range of dosage. Thus, the usefulness of the compound will be correspondingly limited, even though the drug is inherently capable of producing a greater effect. Another example of differences in maximum effect may be found in the analgesic effects of morphine and aspirin. Morphine has sufficient efficacy to provide relief from intense pain that aspirin, even at massive doses, is incapable of relieving. Note that potency and maximum effect of the drug are two separate considerations and, although one compound may be less potent than another, it may still be capable of exerting a greater maximal effect.

VARIABILITY

The final factor to be considered in a dose-response curve is variability. The dose of a drug that will produce a given response in a number of animals will vary considerably. Figure V.4 illustrates a Gaussian (bell-shaped) distribution of drug variability in a population of animals. Note that, although the *average* dose required to elicit a given response in this population of animals may be easily calculated (illustrated by the dotted line), some animals will respond to drug at a dose very much lower than the average and some animals will not respond until extremely large doses have been administered. Because of this variation in susceptibility to drug, it is *extremely important* that the dose of any drug be individualized. Generalizations about "average doses" are risky at best. This Gaussian distribution, however, allows us to estimate the dose of the drug that will produce the desired effect in 50 percent of the subjects. This dose is considered to

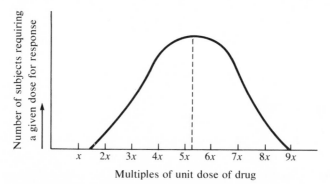

Figure V.4. Biological variation in susceptibility to drugs. This curve is a Gaussian distribution, with the dose of drug plotted against the number of subjects requiring a given dose for a given response to occur. Note that, for a given response, some individuals will require only a small amount of the drug while others will require much more than what is considered normal.

be the ED_{50} for the drug (the effective dose for 50 percent of the subjects).

Closely related to the ED_{50} is the LD_{50} (lethal dose for 50 percent of the subjects). The LD_{50} is calculated exactly like the ED_{50} except that the dose of the drug is plotted against the number of subjects (usually mice) that die following various doses of the compound. Pharmacologists feel that delineation of both the ED_{50} and LD_{50} is necessary for public safety in order to prevent accidental drug-induced deaths in humans. Both the ED_{50} and the LD_{50} are usually determined in laboratory mice and the ratio of the LD_{50} to the ED_{50} is an index of the relative *safety* of the drug. The higher the ratio, the greater the difference between the lethal and effective doses of the compound.

The relation between the ED_{50} and the LD_{50} for a depressant drug is illustrated in Figure V.5, in which two dose-response curves are shown: the one on the left illustrates the dose of drug necessary to induce sleep in the population of mice and the one on the right illustrates the dose of drug necessary to kill a similar population. If one extrapolates across the 50 percent point (dotted lines), and determines the doses necessary to induce sleep in 50 percent and death in another 50 percent, one could determine a ratio between the median toxic dose and the median effective dose ($LD_{50}:ED_{50}$). In this case, the ratio would be 100:10, or 10. This figure is referred to as the *therapeutic index* of the drug—that is, the dose necessary to kill 50 percent of the mice is 10 times that necessary to induce sleep in 50 percent of the animals. This may sound like a rather large margin, but note the 50 mg point on the abscissa. It may be observed that, at the dose of 50 mg, 95 percent of the mice would be put to sleep while 5 percent of the mice would die. This overlap demonstrates the diffi-

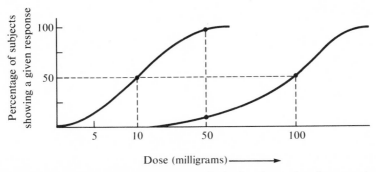

Figure V.5. Two dose-response curves. *Left*, the dose of a drug required to induce a given response. *Right*, the lethal dose of the compound.

culty encountered in assessing the relative safety of drugs for use in large populations and serves as an excellent example of biological variation in individual response to drugs. With this particular compound, a dose could not be administered that would guarantee that 100 percent of the mice would sleep and none would die.

Since the ED_{50} and LD_{50} refer to the means of a population's response to a drug and since these terms do not account for biological variations on the tails of the curves, it has been suggested by some pharmacologists that a more meaningful index of a drug's safety would be a ratio of the lethal dose for 1 percent of the population to the effective dose for 99 percent of the population ($LD_1:ED_{99}$). A pharmacologist would determine the dose that would be effective for 99 percent of the mice and the dose that would be lethal to only 1 percent of the mice. A sedative drug with a $LD_1:ED_{99}$ of 1 would be a safer compound than the drug illustrated in Figure V.5. Thus, these therapeutic ratios offer an index of the relative *safety* of a compound.

It is important to note, however, that a drug does not have a single therapeutic index, but many, because drugs exert more than one effect. Ideally, a therapeutic ratio should be drawn for each observed effect of the drug. For example, the margin of safety for aspirin for relief of headache is greater than its margin of safety for relief of the pain of arthritis since much higher therapeutic doses are used for arthritic pain than for simple headache. The use of such indices obtained from data in laboratory mice is limited. A drug might be found in mice to have an adequate margin of safety for the great majority of patients. But these therapeutic indices seldom consider the patient who for some reason (such as allergy) will exhibit an unusual and unexpected response to the drug. It is important for consumers to realize that, within tolerable limits, a risk/benefit ratio can be calculated for all drugs.

Glossary

Absorption, drug—mechanisms by which a drug reaches the bloodstream from the skin, lungs, stomach, intestinal tract, or muscle.

Abstinence syndrome—a state of altered behavior observed following cessation of drug administration.

Acetylcholine (ACh)—a neurotransmitter in the central and peripheral nervous systems.

Additive effect—an increased effect observed when two drugs having similar biological actions are administered. The net effect is the sum of the independent effects exerted by each drug.

Administration, drug—procedures through which a drug gains entrance into the body (oral administration of tablets or liquids, inhalation of powders, injection of sterile liquids, etc.).

Alcohol (ethyl alcohol, ethanol)—a widely used sedative-hypnotic drug.

Aldehyde dehydrogenase—an enzyme that carries out a specific step in alcohol metabolism: the metabolism of acetaldehyde to acetate. This enzyme may be blocked by the drug disulfiram (Antabuse).

Amphetamine—a behavioral stimulant.

Anesthetic drug—a sedative-hypnotic compound used primarily in doses capable of inducing a state of general anesthesia involving both loss of sensation and loss of consciousness.

Antianxiety agent—a sedative-hypnotic compound used in subhypnotic doses.

Antipsychotic drugs—a class of psychoactive drugs all of which have the ability to calm psychotic states and make the psychotic patient more manageable.

Ascending reticular activating system (ARAS)—a network of neurons in the brainstem thought to function in arousal mechanisms.

Barbiturate—a class of chemically related sedative-hypnotic compounds all of which share a characteristic 6-membered ring structure.

Benzodiazepine—a class of chemically related sedative-hypnotic agents of which chlordiazepoxide (Librium) and diazepam (Valium) are examples.

Brain syndrome, organic—pattern of behavior induced when neurons are either reversibly depressed or irreversibly destroyed. Behavior is characterized by clouded sensorium; disorientation; shallow and labile affect; and impaired memory, intellectual function, insight, and judgment.

Bufotenine—a psychoactive drug found in cohoba snuff, the skin and parotid gland of the toad, and in small amounts in the mushroom *Amanita muscaria*.

Caffeine—a behavioral and general cellular stimulant found in coffee, tea, cola drinks, and chocolate.

Chlordiazepoxide (Librium)—a benzodiazepine, sedative-hypnotic drug.

Chlorpromazine (Thorazine)—a phenothiazine, antipsychotic drug.

Clomiphene (Clomid)—an ovulation-inducing agent thought to act by blocking the inhibitory (negative-feedback) effect that estrogens exert on the hypothalamus.

Cocaine—a behavioral stimulant.

Codeine—a sedative and pain-relieving agent found in opium, structurally related to morphine but less potent, and constituting approximately 0.5 percent of the opium extract.

Cross dependence—a condition in which one drug can prevent the withdrawal symptoms associated with physical dependence on a different drug.

Cross tolerance—a condition in which tolerance of one drug results in a lessened response to another drug.

Delirium tremens (D.T.s, "rum fits")—a syndrome of tremulousness, with hallucinations, psychomotor agitation, confusion and disorientation, sleep disorders, and other associated discomforts, lasting several days after alcohol withdrawal.

Dependency, drug—state in which the use of a drug is necessary for either physical or psychological well-being.

Diisopropyl fluorophosphate (DFP)—an irreversible acetylcholinesterase (AChE) inhibitor.

Diazepam (Valium)—a benzodiazepine, antianxiety drug.

Dicarbamates—a class of chemically related sedative-hypnotic agents of which meprobamate (Equanil, Miltown) is an example.

Diethylstilbestrol—a synthetically produced estrogen occasionally used in high doses as a postcoital contraceptive.

Dimethyltryptamine (DMT)—a psychedelic drug found in many South American snuffs, such as yopo (prepared from the beans of the tree *Piptadenia peregrina*).

Disinhibition—a physiologic state within the central nervous system characterized by decreased activity of inhibitory synapses, which results in a net excess of excitatory activity.

Drug—any chemical substance used for its effects on bodily processes.

Drug interaction—the modification of the action of one drug by the concurrent or prior administration of another drug.

Drug misuse—the use of any drug (legal or illegal) for a medical or recreational purpose when other alternatives are available, practical, or warranted, or when drug use endangers either the user or others with whom he may interact.

Drug receptor—the specific molecular substance in the body with which a given drug interacts in order to produce its effect.

Drug tolerance—a state of progressively decreased responsiveness to a drug.

Enzyme induction—the increased production of drug-metabolizing enzymes in the liver stimulated by certain drugs, such that use of these drugs increases the rate at which the body can metabolize them. It is one mechanism by which pharmacological tolerance is produced.

Estrogen—a body hormone secreted primarily from the ovaries of females in response to stimulation by folicle-stimulating hormone (FSH) from the pituitary gland.

Haloperidol (Haldol)—an antipsychotic drug chemically classified as a butyrophenone.

Harmine—a psychedelic agent obtained from the seeds of *Peganum harmala*.

Hashish—an extract of the hemp plant *(Cannabis sativa)* with a higher concentration of THC than marijuana.

Heroin—a semisynthetic opiate produced by a chemical modification of morphine.

Ketamine (Ketalar)—a psychedelic surgical anesthetic.

Lithium—an alkalai metal effective in the treatment of mania and depression.

Lysergic acid diethylamide (LSD)—a semisynthetic psychedelic drug.

Major tranquilizer (antipsychotic tranquilizer)—a drug used in the treatment of psychotic states.

MAO inhibitor—a drug that inhibits the activity of the enzyme monoamine oxidase.

Marijuana—a mixture of the crushed leaves, flowers, and small branches of both male and female individuals of the hemp plant *(Cannabis sativa)*.

Meperidine (Demerol)—a synthetically produced opiate narcotic.

Meprobamate (Equanil)—a sedative-hypnotic agent frequently used as an antianxiety drug.

Mescaline—a psychedelic drug extracted from the peyote cactus *(Lophophora williamsii)*.

Methadone (Dolophine)—a synthetically produced opiate narcotic.

Methaqualone—a sedative-hypnotic compound of relatively low potency.

Methylphenidate (Ritalin)—a CNS stimulant chemically and pharmacologically related to amphetamine.

Monoamine oxidase (MAO)—an enzyme capable of metabolizing norepinephrine, dopamine, and serotonin to inactive products.

Minor tranquilizer—any sedative-hypnotic drug promoted primarily for use in the treatment of anxiety.

Morphine—the major sedative and pain-relieving drug found in opium, being approximately 10 percent of the crude opium exudate.

Muscarine—a drug extracted from the mushroom *Amanita muscaria* that directly stimulates acetylcholine receptors.

Myristicin—a psychedelic agent obtained from nutmeg and mace.

Nicotine—a behavioral stimulant found in tobacco.

Norepinephrine (NE)—a synaptic transmitter in both the central and peripheral nervous systems.

Ololiuqui—a psychedelic drug obtained from the seeds of the morning glory.

Opiate—any natural or synthetic drug that exerts actions on the body similar to those induced by morphine, the major pain-relieving agent obtained from the opium poppy *(Papaver somniferum)*.

Opiate narcotic—a drug that has both sedative and analgesic actions.

Opium—a crude resinous exudate from the opium poppy.

Parkinson's disease—a disorder of the motor system characterized by involuntary movements, tremor, and weakness.

Pentylenetetrazol (Metrazol)—a convulsant drug.

Pharmacology—the branch of science that deals with the study of drugs and their actions on living systems.

Phencyclidine (Sernyl)—a psychedelic surgical anesthetic.

Phenothiazine—a class of chemically related compounds useful in the treatment of psychosis.

Physical dependence—a state in which the presence of a drug is required in order for an individual to function normally. Such a state is revealed by withdrawing the drug and noting the occurrence of withdrawal symptoms (abstinence syndrome). Characteristically, withdrawal symptoms can be terminated by readministration of the drug.

Physostigmine—an acetylcholinesterase (AChE) inhibitor.

Picrotoxin—a convulsant drug.

Placebo—a pharmacologically inert substance that may elicit a significant reaction largely because of the mental "set" of the patient or the physical setting in which the drug is taken.

Potency—a measure of drug activity expressed in terms of the amount required to produce an effect of given intensity. Potency varies inversely with the amount of drug required to produce this effect—that is, the more potent the drug, the lower the amount required to produce the effect.

Progesterone—a hormone secreted from the ovaries in response to stimulation by luteinizing hormone (LH) from the pituitary gland.

Progestins—a group of synthetically produced progesterones, most frequently found in oral contraceptive tablets.

Psilocybin—a psychoactive drug obtained from the Mexican mushroom *Psilocybe mexicana*.

Psychoactive drug—any chemical substance that alters mood or behavior as a result of alterations in the functioning of the brain.

Psychological dependence—a compulsion to use a drug for its pleasurable effects. Such dependence may lead to a compulsion to misuse a drug.

Psychedelic drug—any drug with the ability to alter sensory perception.

Reserpine (Serpasil)—an antipsychotic drug.

Risk/benefit ratio—an arbitrary assessment of the risks and benefits that may accrue from administration of a drug.

Sedative-hypnotic drug—any chemical substance that exerts a non-selective general depressant action upon the central nervous system.

Seretonin (5-hydroxtryptamine, 5-HT)—a synaptic transmitter both in the brain and in the peripheral nervous system.

Side effect—any drug-induced effect that accompanies the primary effect for which the drug was administered.

Stimulant—any drug that increases behavioral activity.

Strychnine—a convulsant drug.

Teratogen—any chemical substance that may induce abnormalities of fetal development.

Testosterone—a hormone secreted from the testes that is responsible for the distinguishing characteristics of the male.

Tetrahydrocannabinol (THC)—a major psychoactive agent found in marijuana, hashish, and other preparations of hemp *(Cannabis sativa)*.

Tolerance, drug—state of progressively decreasing responsiveness to a drug.

Toxic effect—any drug-induced effect that is either temporarily or permanently deleterious to any organ or system of an animal or patient to which the drug is administered. Drug toxicity includes both the relatively minor side effects that invariably accompany drug administration and the more serious and unexpected manifestations that occur in only a small percentage of individuals taking a drug.

Bibliography

TEXTBOOKS OF PHARMACOLOGY

Bevan, J. A. *Essentials of Pharmacology,* 2d ed. New York: Harper & Row, 1976.

DiPalma, J. R. *Basic Pharmacology in Medicine.* New York: McGraw-Hill, 1976.

Goldstein, A., L. Aronow, and S. M. Kalman. *Principles of Drug Action,* 2d ed. New York: Harper & Row, 1974.

Goodman, L. S., and A. Gilman, eds. *The Pharmacological Basis of Therapeutics,* 4th ed., 5th ed. New York: Macmillan, 1970, 1975. (4th edition has information on psychedelic drugs not found in newer edition.)

Goth, A. *Medical Pharmacology,* 7th ed. St. Louis: C. V. Mosby, 1975.

LaDu, B. N., H. G. Mandel, and E. L. Way. *Fundamentals of Drug Metabolism and Drug Disposition.* Baltimore: Williams and Wilkins, 1971.

273

Meyers, F. H., E. Jawetz, and A. Goldfien. *Review of Medical Pharma-cology,* 5th ed. Los Altos, Calif: Lange Medical Publications, 1976.

ALCOHOL AND ALCOHOLISM

Cahn, *The Treatment of Alcoholics: An Evaluation Study.* New York: Oxford University Press, 1970.

Israel, Y., and J. Mardones. *The Biological Basis of Alcoholism.* New York: Wiley-Interscience, 1971.

Jellinek, E. M. *The Disease Concept of Alcoholism.* New Haven, Conn.: Hillhouse Press, 1960.

Jones, K. L., L. W. Shainberg, and C. O. Byer. *Drugs and Alcohol.* New York: Harper & Row, 1969.

Ludwig, A. M., J. Levine, and L. H. Stark. *LSD and Alcoholism: A Clini-cal Study of Treatment Efficacy.* Springfield, Ill.: C. C. Thomas, 1970.

Mann, M. *New Primer on Alcoholism,* 2d ed. New York: Holt, Rinehart and Winston, 1968.

Mello, N. K. "Some Aspects of the Behavioral Pharmacology of Alcohol." In *Psychopharmacology: A Review of Progress, 1957–1967,* D. H. Efron, ed. Washington, D.C.: U.S. Government Printing Office, 1968.

Mendelson, J. H. "The Biochemical Pharmacology of Alcohol." In *Psy-chopharmacology: A Review of Progress, 1957–1967,* D. H. Ef-ron, ed. Washington, D.C.: U.S. Government Printing Office, 1968.

Milner, J. *Drugs and Driving* (Monographs on Drugs, vol. 1). Basel: S. Karger, 1972.

National Institute on Alcohol Abuse and Alcoholism. *Facts About Alcohol and Alcoholism.* DNEW Publication no. (ADM) 75–31. Washington, D.C.: U.S. Government Printing Office, 1974.

Pattison, E. M. "The Rehabilitation of the Chronic Alcoholic." Pp. 587–658 in *The Biology of Alcoholism,* vol. 3, B. Kissin and H. Begletier, eds. New York: Plenum Press, 1974.

Pattison, E. M., M. B. Sobell, and L. C. Sobell. *Emerging Concepts of Alcohol Dependence.* New York: Springer-Verlag, 1977.

Seixas, F. A., K. Williams, and S. Eggleston, eds. "Medical Consequences of Alcoholism," *Annals of the New York Academy of Sciences* 252 (25 April 1975).

Sobell, M.B., and L. C. Sobell, *Individualized Behavioral Treatment of Alcohol Problems.* New York: Plenum Press, 1977.

U.S. Department of Health, Education, and Welfare. *Second Special Report to the United States Congress on Alcohol and Health*. Washington, D.C.: U.S. Government Printing Office, 1974.

HEROIN AND OPIATE NARCOTICS

Brecher, E. M., and *Consumer Reports* editors. *Licit and Illicit Drugs: The Consumers Union Report on Narcotics, Stimulants, Depressants, Inhalants, Hallucinogens, and Marihuana—Including Caffeine, Nicotine, and Alcohol*. Mount Vernon, N.Y.: Consumers Union, 1972.

Chien, I., D. L. Gerard, R. S. Lee, and E. Rosenfeld. *The Road to H: Narcotics, Delinquency, and Social Policy*. New York: Basic Books, 1964.

DeLong, J. V. "Treatment and Rehabilitation." In *Dealing with Drug Abuse—A Report to the Ford Foundation,* prepared by the Drug Abuse Survey Project, P. M. Wald and P. B. Hutt, cochairmen. New York: Praeger, 1972.

Jaffee, J. H. "Narcotic Analgesics and Antagonists." In *The Pharmacological Basis of Therapeutics,* 5th ed., L. S. Goodman and A. Gilman, eds. New York: Macmillan, 1975.

Smith, D. E., and G. R. Gay. *It's So Good, Don't Even Try It Once: Heroin in Perspective*. Englewood Cliffs, N.J.: Prentice-Hall, 1972.

ANTIPSYCHOTIC TRANQUILIZERS

Clark, W. G., and J. del Giudice. *Principles of Psychopharmacology*. New York: Academic Press, 1970.

Klawans, H. L., ed. *Clinical Pharmacology,* vol. 1. New York: Raven Press, 1976.

Longo, V. G. *Neuropharmacology and Behavior*. San Francisco: W. H. Freeman, 1972.

Schou, M. "Pharmacology and Toxicology of Lithium." Pp. 231–43 in *Annual Review of Pharmacology and Toxicology,* vol. 16, H. W. Elliott, ed. Palo Alto, Calif.: Annual Reviews, 1976.

Simpson, L. L., ed. *Drug Treatment of Mental Disorders*. New York: Raven Press, 1976.

Snider, S. H., S. P. Banerjee, H. I. Yamamura, and D. Greenberg. "Drugs, Neurotransmitters, and Schizophrenia," *Science* 184 (24 June 1974): 1243–53.

Von Brucke, F. T., O. Hornykiewicz, and E. B. Sigg. *The Pharmacology of Psychotherapeutic Drugs*. New York: Springer-Verlag, 1969.

CANNABIS

Government Reports

Cannabis: A Report of the Commission of Inquiry into the Non-medical Use of Drugs. Gerald LeDain, chairman. Ottawa: Information Canada, 1972.

Interim Report of the Commission of Inquiry into the Non-medical Use of Drugs. Gerald LeDain, chairman. Ottawa: Information Canada, 1970.

National Commission on Marihuana and Drug Abuse, Raymond P. Shafer, chairman. *Drug Use in America: The Problem in Perspective*. Washington, D.C.: U.S. Government Printing Office, 1973.

National Commission on Marihuana and Drug Abuse, Raymond P. Shafer, chairman. *Marihuana: A Signal of Misunderstanding*. New York: New American Library, 1972.

The President's Commission on Law Enforcement and Administration of Justice. *Task Force Report: Narcotics and Drug Abuse*. Washington, D.C.: U.S. Government Printing Office, 1967.

Secretary of Health, Education, and Welfare. *Marihuana and Health: Fourth Annual Report to the U.S. Congress*. Washington, D.C.: U.S. Government Printing Office, 1974.

Other Recommended References

Braude, M. C. and S. S. Szara, eds. *Pharmacology of Marihuana* (2 vols.) New York: Raven Press, 1976.

Brecher, E. M., and *Consumer Reports* editors. *Licit and Illicit Drugs: The Consumers Union Report on Narcotics, Stimulants, Depressants, Inhalants, Hallucinogens, and Marihuana—Including Caffeine, Nicotine, and Alcohol*. Mount Vernon, N.Y.: Consumers Union, 1972.

Brecher, E. M., and *Consumer Reports* editors. "Marijuana: The Health Questions," *Consumer Reports* 40 (March 1975): 143–49.

Dornbush, R. L., A. M. Freedman, and M. Fink, eds. "Chronic Cannabis Use," *Annals of the New York Academy of Sciences* 282 (1976): 1–430.

The Indian Hemp Drugs Commission Report, 1893–94. Contained in 7 volumes and 2 supplements. Simla: Government Central Printing Office. Reprinted in 1971 by Johnson Reprint Corp., New York.

Mikuriya, T. H., ed. *Marijuana: Medical Papers, 1839–1972*. Oakland, Calif.: Medi-Comp Press, 1973.

Nahas, G. G. *Marihuana: Deceptive Weed*. New York: Raven Press, 1974.

New York Academy of Sciences. "Marihuana: Chemistry, Pharmacology and Patterns of Social Use," *Annals of the New York Academy of Sciences* 191 (31 December 1971).

The Mayor's Committee on Marihuana. *The Marihuana Problem in the City of New York*. Lancaster, Pa.: The Mayor's Committee on Marihuana, 1944. Reprinted in 1973 by Scarecrow Reprint Corp., Metuchen, N.J., and published under the auspices of the Library of the New York Academy of Medicine.

Paton, W. D. M. "Pharmacology of Marijuana." Pp. 191–220 in *Annual Review of Pharmacology*, vol. 15, H. W. Elliott, ed. Palo Alto, Calif.: Annual Reviews, 1975.

NERVE PHYSIOLOGY AND NEUROANATOMY

Cooper, J. R., F. E. Bloom, and R. H. Roth. *The Biochemical Basis of Neuropharmacology*. New York: Oxford University Press, 1974.

Eccles, J. C. *The Understanding of the Brain*. New York: McGraw-Hill, 1973.

Grossman, S. P. *A Textbook of Physiological Psychology*. New York: John Wiley, 1967.

Isaacson, R. L., R. J. Douglas, J. F. Lubar, and L. W. Schmaltz. *A Primer of Physiological Psychology*. New York: Harper & Row, 1971.

Iverson, S. D., and L. L. Iverson. *Behavioral Pharmacology*. New York: Oxford University Press, 1975.

Netter, Frank H. *The Nervous System* (the Ciba Collection of Medical Illustrations, vol. 1). Summit, N.J.: Ciba Pharmaceutical Products, 1962.

Rech, R. A., and K. W. Moore. *An Introduction to Psychopharmacology*. New York: Raven Press, 1971.

Ruch, P. C., and H. D. Patton. *Physiology and Biophysics*. Philadelphia: Saunders, 1965.

Schmidt, R. F. *Fundamentals of Neurophysiology*. New York: Springer-Verlag, 1975.

Smith, C. G. *Basic Neuroanatomy*. Toronto: University of Toronto Press, 1961.

Stevens, Charles F. *Neurophysiology: A Primer*. New York: John Wiley, 1966.

Thompson, Richard F. *Foundations of Physiologic Psychology*. New York: Harper & Row, 1967.

DRUG EDUCATION

Cornacchia, H., D. Bentel, and D. Smith. *Drugs in the Classroom*. Saint Louis, Mo.: C.V. Mosby, 1973.

The Drug Abuse Survey Project. *Dealing with Drug Abuse: A Report to the Ford Foundation*. New York: Praeger, 1972.

Marin, P., and A. Y. Cohen. *Understanding Drug Use*. New York: Harper & Row, 1971.

National Institute on Drug Abuse. *Doing Drug Education: The Role of the School Teacher*. Washington, D.C.: U.S. Government Printing Office, 1975.

National Institute on Drug Abuse. *Why Evaluate Drug Education? Task Force Report*. Washington, D.C.: U.S. Government Printing Office, 1975.

Sherman, G. P., and W. C. Lubawy. "Development of a Drug Education Training Course for School Teachers," *American Journal of Pharmaceutical Education* 40 (May 1976): 161–64.

Weil, A. *The Natural Mind*. Boston: Houghton Mifflin, 1973.

Index